## DATE DUE

| | | | |
|---|---|---|---|
| 1-10 | | | |
| 5-5-01 | | | |
| MAY 9 2001 | | | |
| | | | |
| | | | |
| | | | |
| | | | |
| | | | |
| | | | |
| | | | |
| | | | |
| | | | |

# Innovations
# in Alcoholism Treatment:
# State of the Art Reviews
# and Their Implications
# for Clinical Practice

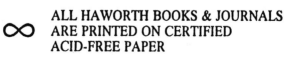

# Innovations in Alcoholism Treatment: State of the Art Reviews and Their Implications for Clinical Practice

Gerard J. Connors, PhD
Editor

The Haworth Press, Inc.
New York · London · Norwood (Australia)

*Innovations in Alcoholism Treatment: State of the Art Reviews and Their Implications for Clinical Practice* has also been published as *Drugs & Society,* Volume 8, Number 1 1993.

The development, preparation, and publication of this work has been undertaken with great care. However, the publisher, employees, editors, and agents of The Haworth Press and all imprints of The Haworth Press, Inc., including The Haworth Medical Press and Pharmaceutical Products Press, are not responsible for any errors contained herein or for consequences that may ensue from use of materials or information contained in this work. Opinions expressed by the author(s) are not necessarily those of The Haworth Press, Inc.

The Haworth Press, Inc., 10 Alice Street, Binghamton, NY 13904-1580 USA

**Library of Congress Cataloging-in-Publication Data**

Innovations in alcoholism treatment: state of the art reviews and their implications for clinical practice/Gerard J. Connors, editor.
    p. cm.
"Published as Drugs & society, v. 8, no. 1, 1993" - T.p, verso.
Includes bibliographical references.
ISBN 1-56024-657-X (acid-free paper)
1. Alcohlism–Treatment. 2. Alcoholism. I. Connors, Gerard Joseph.

RC565.I486 1993                                  93-49064
616.86'106–dc20                                    CIP

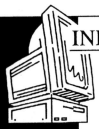

# INDEXING & ABSTRACTING

Contributions to this publication are selectively indexed or abstracted in print, electronic, online, or CD-ROM version(s) of the reference tools and information services listed below. This list is current as of the copyright date of this publication. See the end of this section for additional notes.

- *Abstracts in Anthropology*, Baywood Publishing Company, 26 Austin Avenue, P.O. Box 337, Amityville, NY 11701

- *ALCONARC Database*, Swedish Council for Information on Alcohol and Other Drugs, Box 27302, S-102 54 Stockholm, Sweden

- *Applied Social Sciences Index & Abstracts (ASSIA)*, Bowker-Saur Limited, East Grinstead, East Sussex, RH19 1HH, England

- *Cambridge Scientific Abstracts, Health & Safety Science Abstracts*, Cambridge Information Group, 7200 Wisconsin Avenue #601, Bethesda, MD 20814

- *Child Development Abstracts & Bibliography*, University of Kansas, 2 Bailey Hall, Lawrence, KS 66045

- *Criminal Justice Abstracts*, Willow Tree Press, 15 Washington Street, 4th Floor, Newark, NJ 07102

- *Criminal Justice Periodical Index*, University Microfilms, Inc., 300 North Zeeb Road, Ann Arbor, MI 48106

- *Excerpta Medica/Electronic Publishing Division*, Elsevier Science Publishers, 655 Avenue of the Americas, New York, NY 10010

(continued)

- *Human Resources Abstracts*, Sage Publications, Inc., 2455 Teller Road, Newbury Park, CA 91320

- *Index to Periodical Articles Related to Law*, University of Texas, 727 East 26th Street, Austin, TX 78705

- *International Pharmaceutical Abstracts*, American Society of Hospital Pharmacists, 7272 Wisconsin Avenue, Bethesda, MD 20814

- *International Political Science Abstracts*, 27 Rue Saint-Guillaume, F75337 Paris, Cedex 07, France

- *Inventory of Marriage and Family Literature (online and hard copy)*, National Council on Family Relations, 3989 Central Avenue NE, Suite 550, Minneapolis, MN 55421

- *Medication Use STudies (MUST) DATABASE*, School of Pharmacy, The University of Mississippi, University, MS 38677

- *Mental Health Abstracts (online through DIALOG)*, IFI/Plenum Data Company, 3202 Kirkwood Highway, Wilmington, DE 19808

- *NIAAA Alcohol and Alcohol Problems Science Database (ETOH)*, National Institute on Alcohol Abuse and Alcoholism, 1400 Eye Street NW, Suite 600, Washington, DC 20005

- *Personnel Management Abstracts*, 704 Island Lake Road, Chelsea, MI 48118

- *Psychological Abstracts (PsycINFO)*, American Psychological Association, P.O. Box 91600, Washington, DC 20090-1600

- *Public Affairs Information Bulletin (PAIS)*, Public Affairs Information Service, Inc., 521 West 43rd Street, New York, NY 10036-4396

(continued)

- *Referativnyi Zhurnal (Abstracts Journal of the Institute of Scientific Information of the Republic of Russia)*, The Institute of Scientific Information, Baltijskaja ul., 14, Moscow A-219, Republic of Russia

- *Sage Family Studies Abstracts*, Sage Publications, Inc., 2455 Teller Road, Newbury Park, CA 91320

- *Social Planning/Policy & Development Abstracts (SOPODA)*, Sociological Abstracts, Inc., P.O. Box 22206, San Diego, CA 92192-0206

- *Social Service Abstracts*, Department of Health, Room G12, Wellington House, 133-135 Waterloo Road, London SE1 8UG, England

- *Social Work Research & Abstracts*, National Association of Social Workers, 750 First Street NW, 8th Floor, Washington, DC 20002

- *Sociological Abstracts (SA)*, Sociological Abstracts, Inc., P.O. Box 22206, San Diego, CA 92192-0206

- *SOMED (social medicine) Database*, Institute fur Dokumentation, Postfach 20 10 12, D-4800 Bielefeld 1, Germany

- *Sport Database/Discus*, Sport Information Resource Center, 1600 James Naismith Drive, Suite 107, Gloucester, Ontario K1B 5N4, Canada

- *The Brown University Digest of Addiction Theory and Application (Data Newsletter)*, Project Cork Institute, Dartmouth Medical School, 14 S. Main Street, Suite 2F Hanover NH 03755-2015

- *Urban Affairs Abstracts*, National League of Cities, 1301 Pennsylvania Avenue NW, Washington, DC 20004

# SPECIAL BIBLIOGRAPHIC NOTES

*related to indexing, abstracting, and library access services*

❑ indexing/abstracting services in this list will also cover material in the "separate" that is co-published simultaneously with Haworth's special thematic journal issue or DocuSerial. Indexing/abstracting usually covers material at the article/chapter level.

❑ monographic co-editions are intended for either non-subscribers or libraries which intend to purchase a second copy for their circulating collections.

❑ monographic co-editions are reported to all jobbers/wholesalers/approval plans. The source journal is listed as the "series" to assist the prevention of duplicate purchasing in the same manner utilized for books-in-series.

❑ to facilitate user/access services all indexing/abstracting services are encouraged to utilize the co-indexing entry note indicated at the bottom of the first page of each article/chapter/contribution.

❑ this is intended to assist a library user of any reference tool (whether print, electronic, online, or CD-ROM) to locate the monographic version if the library has purchased this version but not a subscription to the source journal.

❑ individual articles/chapters in any Haworth publication are also available through the Haworth Document Delivery Services (HDDS).

# Innovations in Alcoholism Treatment: State of the Art Reviews and Their Implications for Clinical Practice

## CONTENTS

**Foreword**                                                                    xiii

**An Overview and Critique of Advances in the Treatment of Alcohol Use Disorders**                                      1
*James R. McKay*
*Stephen A. Maisto*

Efficacy of Standard Treatments for Alcoholism             3
Brief Interventions                                                          5
Cost Effectiveness of Alcoholism Treatments              6
Patient-Treatment Matching                                            7
Treatment Process                                                         10
Relapse Prevention                                                        11
Effectiveness of Self-Help Groups                              12
Treatment of Dual-Diagnosis Alcoholics                     13
Pharmacotherapy                                                           17
Discussion                                                                     18

**Recent Developments in Detection and Biological Indicators of Alcoholism**                                       31
*Arthur W. K. Chan, PhD*

Introduction                                                                   31
Screening Questionnaires                                             33
Biochemical Indicators                                                  39
Conclusions                                                                   53

**Modern Disease Models of Alcoholism and Other Chemical Dependencies: The New Biopsychosocial Models**     **69**
*John Wallace*

The Disease Concept in Historical Perspective     71
Emerging Criticism     73
The Need for Revision: The New Biopsychosocial Models     76
Utilizing Biopsychosocial Models in Chemical Dependence
    Treatment     78
Psychological Factors and Biopsychosocial Models     82
Sociocultural Surrounds     83
The New Disease Models: Is There Really an Argument?     85


**Sociocultural Aspects of Alcohol Use and Abuse: Ethnicity and Gender**     **89**
*R. Lorraine Collins*

Ethnicity as a Sociocultural Factor in Alcohol Research     90
Gender as a Sociocultural Factor in Alcohol Research     95
Overview of Research on the Prevalence of Alcohol Abuse     96
Overview of Research on the Prevention of Alcohol Abuse     99
Overview of Research on the Treatment of Alcohol Abuse     105
Recommendations for Future Research on Treatment
    for Alcohol Abuse     107
Conclusions     110


**Drinking Moderation Training as a Contemporary Therapeutic Approach**     **117**
*Gerard J. Connors*

Introduction     118
Historical Overview     118
Current Status Regarding Drinking Moderation
    Treatments     124
Some Directions for Future Research     128
Conclusions     130

# ABOUT THE EDITOR

**Gerard J. Connors, PhD,** is Senior Research Scientist at the Research Institute on Addictions in Buffalo, New York, and holds appointments with the Department of Psychology at the State University of New York at Buffalo and with the Department of Psychiatry at the State University of New York Medical School at Buffalo. His major clinical research interests include treatment of alcoholism and other substance abuse, treatment outcome research, early intervention, and relapse prevention. Co-author of a textbook on drug use and misuse, Dr. Connors has published a number of book chapters and over fifty articles in refereed journals. Currently, he is collaborating on several clinical research projects funded by the National Institute on Alcohol Abuse and Alcoholism. Dr. Connors is a licensed psychologist and holds Diplomate status from the American Board of Professional Psychology.

# Foreword

Researchers and clinicians in the alcohol field are alike in that they lead hectic professional lives. Their daily routines generally do not afford the luxury of thoughtfully keeping abreast of the vast amount of diverse yet relevant research being conducted in the alcohol field. Indeed, it often is difficult to find time to sit back and consolidate one's thoughts and impressions about a particular area of research. It was largely for that reason that the present volume was conceived. More specifically, this volume was developed to provide state-of-the-art reviews and perspectives on several important current areas of research in the field of alcoholism. In this regard, each of the articles includes a summary and synthesis of current research. Importantly, the articles include commentaries on the clinical and research implications of their topics and indicate directions for future research. As such, the papers in this volume will provide information on where we have been, where we now are, and where we may be heading in terms of important clinical research issues.

In the opening article, entitled "An Overview and Critique of Advances in the Treatment of Alcohol Use Disorders," James McKay and Stephen Maisto review recent developments in the arena of alcoholism treatment research. The host of topics addressed includes patient-treatment matching, treatment process variables, the cost-effectiveness of alcoholism treatment, the efficacy of self-help groups, treatment of dual-diagnosis alcoholics, and pharmacotherapy. Recent research on each of these topics is reviewed and clinical implications discussed. McKay and Maisto also

[Haworth co-indexing entry note]: "Foreword," Gerard J. Connors. Co-published simultaneously in *Drugs & Society* (The Haworth Press, Inc.) Vol. 8, No. 1, 1993, pp. xiii-xv; and: *Innovations in Alcoholism Treatment: State of the Art Reviews and Their Implications for Clinical Practice* (ed: Gerard J. Connors) The Haworth Press, Inc., 1993, pp. xiii-xv. Multiple copies of this article/chapter may be purchased from The Haworth Document Delivery Center [1-800-3-HAWORTH; 9:00 a.m. - 5:00 p.m. (EST)].

identify issues surrounding these topics that remain unresolved. They close with suggestions regarding future research.

Arthur Chan, in his article "Recent Developments in Detection and Biological Indicators of Alcoholism," presents a comprehensive and integrated review of contemporary research on the identification of alcohol use disorders. He begins with a presentation on screening questionnaires that can be used productively and efficiently in the identification of alcohol abusers. Such instruments can be used in concert with laboratory indicators of excessive drinking. In this regard, Chan reviews the latest developments in the area of biological indicators of alcoholism. He covers as well current research on biological indicators of vulnerability ("trait markers") for developing alcohol use problems. An emphasis throughout Chan's article is the need to implement detection mechanisms, whether they be questionnaire, laboratory, or both, in those settings most likely to permit early identification of and intervention with persons experiencing alcohol use disorders.

The third article, by John Wallace, is entitled "Modern Disease Models of Alcoholism and Other Chemical Dependencies: The New Biopsychosocial Models." Wallace addresses the topic of contemporary disease models of alcoholism and other chemical dependencies. He notes that the disease concept has had a profound impact on the chemical dependency field. After providing a historical perspective on the disease concept, Wallace identifies and discusses the criticisms that have been raised regarding the disease concept. In doing so he lays groundwork for outlining some revisions to the disease concept in order to keep it abreast of ongoing research and clinical observations. An emphasis in his article is on a biopsychosocial model of addictions in recognition of the significant roles played by biological, behavioral, cognitive, psychological, and sociocultural factors in the development and maintenance of addictive behaviors. The advantages of a biopsychosocial model are numerous, and they are described by Wallace, who also provides a discussion of the clinical implications of such an approach.

In the fourth article, "Sociocultural Aspects of Alcohol Use and Abuse: Ethnicity and Gender," Lorraine Collins first provides a discussion on ethnicity and gender as sociocultural variables that require attention in the conduct of alcohol research. She then presents a comprehensive and thoughtful review of research on ethnicity and gender as they relate to the prevalence rates of alcohol and substance use/abuse, the development of primary prevention strategies, and the delivery of effective treatment interventions. In terms of ethnicity, Collins focuses in particular on the four major non-European ethnic groups in the United States: African-Americans, American Indians, Asian-Americans, and Latinos.

The final article, "Drinking Moderation Training as a Contemporary Therapeutic Approach," reviews the issue of moderate drinking interventions with alcohol abusers. The article opens with a historical overview of what often has been a controversial topic. The assessment of the current status of drinking moderation treatments in this article is then focused on two topics: the validity of moderate drinking treatment approaches as a contemporary therapeutic strategy and whether research in this area has helped or hindered progress in the treatment of alcohol problems. It is argued in this paper that moderate drinking interventions are a viable treatment strategy for some alcohol abusers and that research on moderate drinking has fostered progress in the treatment of alcohol problems. The article also offers directions for future research on this topic.

The volume as a whole covers a range of topics with direct relevance to understanding the nature of alcohol use disorders and developing strategies for identification and intervention. While each of the authors identifies shortcomings in our present knowledge and methodologies, they just as importantly emphasize the numerous advances that are occurring throughout the field. It is anticipated that the reviews and commentaries provided by these authors will inform the field in ways that are useful to researchers and clinicians alike.

*Gerard J. Connors*

# An Overview and Critique of Advances in the Treatment of Alcohol Use Disorders

James R. McKay
Stephen A. Maisto

SUMMARY. This article reviews recent developments in the field of alcoholism treatment research. The following major topics are addressed: the relative efficacy and cost-effectiveness of various treatment approaches, the use of brief interventions, the identification of patient-treatment matches and treatment processes that predict better outcomes, the efficacy of self-help groups, relapse prevention, the treatment of dual-diagnosis alcoholics, and pharmacotherapy. Under-studied and unresolved issues are identified and discussed, and suggestions are made concerning future research.

Although much attention has been paid in recent years to the problems associated with drug abuse, alcohol use disorders continue to be the most pervasive form of substance abuse in the United States, other than tobacco use (Institute of Medicine, 1990). Fur-

James R. McKay is affiliated with the University of Pennsylvania, Treatment Research Center, 3900 Chestnut Street, Philadelphia, PA 19104. Stephen A. Maisto is affiliated with the Brockton VAMC (116B), 940 Belmont St., Brockton MA, 02401, and Brown University.

This work was supported in part by the National Institute of Drug Abuse Center Grant DA05186, Charles O'Brien, MD, PhD, Principal Investigator.
Address correspondence to James R. McKay.

[Haworth co-indexing entry note]: "An Overview and Critique of Advances in the Treatment of Alcohol Use Disorders," McKay, James R., and Stephen A. Maisto. Co-published simultaneously in *Drugs & Society* (The Haworth Press, Inc.) Vol. 8, No. 1, 1993, pp. 1-29; and: *Innovations in Alcoholism Treatment: State of the Art Reviews and Their Implications for Clinical Practice* (ed: Gerard J. Connors) The Haworth Press, Inc., 1993, pp. 1-29. Multiple copies of this article/chapter may be purchased from The Haworth Document Delivery Center [1-800-3-HAWORTH; 9:00 a.m. - 5:00 p.m. (EST)].

thermore, epidemiological studies have found alcohol abuse or dependence to be the most common psychiatric disorder among men and in the top five among women (Robins et al., 1984; Robins, Helzer, Przybeck, & Reiger, 1988). Over the last two decades, there have been substantial increases in the number of approaches used to treat alcohol use disorders (Institute of Medicine, 1990; Miller & Hester, 1986a). During the same period, the development of new instruments to measure drinking and related problems, such as the Time Line Follow-Back (Sobell, Maisto, Sobell, & Cooper, 1979) and the Addiction Severity Index (McLellan, Luborsky, Woody, & O'Brien, 1980), has increased the reliability and validity of outcome assessments and has led to improvements in the quality of treatment outcome research.

There is now considerable evidence that most alcohol abusers drink less frequently and consume less alcohol when they do drink after receiving alcoholism treatment, compared to their pretreatment drinking behavior (McLellan, Luborsky, O'Brien, Barr, & Evans, 1986; McKay, Murphy, & Longabaugh, 1991; Miller & Hester, 1986a; Moos, Finney, & Cronkite, 1990). Treatment also has been shown to bring about improvements in family functioning, marital satisfaction, and psychiatric impairments (McCrady et al., 1986; McLellan, Woody, Luborsky, O'Brien, & Druley, 1983; O'Farrell, Cutter, & Floyd, 1985). Although improvements following alcoholism treatment are at least in part attributable to nontreatment factors such as patient motivation (Miller, 1986), it is generally accepted that treatment does make a difference, at least in the short run.

In this article, we review selected studies that are relevant to what we view as major topics in alcoholism treatment research: the relative efficacy and cost-effectiveness of various treatment approaches; the use of brief interventions; the identification of patient-treatment matches and treatment processes that predict better outcomes; the efficacy of self-help groups; relapse prevention; the treatment of dual-diagnosis alcoholics; and pharmacotherapy. We then identify and discuss under-studied and unresolved issues in alcoholism treatment research, and make suggestions concerning future research.

## EFFICACY OF STANDARD TREATMENTS
## FOR ALCOHOLISM

In this section, studies that have examined the impact of treatment setting, duration, therapeutic orientation, and the participation of significant others are discussed.

*Treatment Setting.* One of the more thoroughly researched questions in alcoholism treatment is whether inpatient rehabilitation is more effective than treatment carried out on an outpatient basis. Two thorough reviews of over a dozen controlled studies of the effectiveness of inpatient versus non-inpatient treatment have been independently compiled by Longabaugh (1988) and Miller and Hester (1986b). These reviews concluded that for most alcoholics, inpatient treatment was not superior to other settings, such as day treatment, halfway house, or outpatient treatment. In a study just concluded at the University of Pennsylvania, for example, inpatient treatment was actually slightly less effective than day hospital rehabilitation, both for patients who were randomly assigned to treatment conditions and for those who were not (McKay, Alterman, McLellan, & Snider, 1993). There is some evidence, however, that inpatient treatment followed by attendance at AA meetings is more effective than AA alone (Walsh et al., 1991).

*Duration and Intensity of Treatment.* Studies have consistently shown that treatment completion and longer stays in treatment are associated with better drinking outcomes for alcoholic patients, even after controlling for pretreatment drinking severity (McKay, Alterman, McLellan, & Snider, in press a; Moos et al., 1990). However, patients who are randomly assigned to longer stays in residential programs generally do not have better drinking outcomes than those assigned to shorter stays (Longabaugh, 1988).

There is some evidence that comprehensive treatment programs are more effective than less intensive interventions. Patients in a half-way house program that featured daily AA meetings and a work program had better drinking outcomes than matched subjects treated with hospital-based detoxification only (Smith, 1985, 1986). Another comprehensive intervention, the "Community Reinforcement Approach" (CRA), has done extremely well when pitted against other interventions (Azrin, 1976). CRA includes conjoint therapy, job finding training, counseling focused on alcohol-free social and recreational activities, monitored disulfiram, and an alcohol-free social club (Azrin, 1976; Hunt & Azrin, 1973). In a study in which patients were randomly assigned to CRA or a standard hospital treatment program, those getting CRA drank less, spent fewer days away from home, worked more days, and were institutionalized less over a 24 month follow-up (Azrin, 1976). A second controlled study contrasted CRA, disulfiram with a behavioral compliance program, and regular outpatient treatment (Azrin, Sisson, Meyers, & Godley, 1982). Once again, those treated with CRA did substantially better on all outcome measures than those in the other treatment conditions.

*Therapeutic Orientation.* Many therapeutic approaches have been used with alcoholics, including 12-Step based counseling, psychodynamic, and cognitive-behavioral interventions. Holder, Longabaugh, Miller, and Rubonis (1991) recently reviewed the literature on the effectiveness of individual and group psychotherapy with alcoholics. These authors concluded that cognitive-behavioral therapy appeared to have some edge over other therapeutic orientations. Cognitive-behavioral interventions that have been shown to be effective include social skills training (Chaney, 1989) and communication skills training (Monti et al., 1990). However, in one aftercare study, cognitive-behavioral and interactional treatments were equally effective (Cooney, Kadden, Litt, & Getter, 1991; Kadden, Cooney, Getter, & Litt, 1989).

*Participation of Significant Others.* The state of the alcoholic's relationship with family or significant others can be one of the more critical factors in the posttreatment environment (Moos & Moos, 1984). This raises the possibility that conjoint treatment may be particularly effective for alcoholics who are married or living with family members. In controlled studies of marital therapy, behavioral marital therapy (BMT) has fared particularly well (Holder et al., 1991).

For example, O'Farrell et al. (1985) contrasted BMT and interactional marital therapy with a no treatment control group. Both treatment groups showed greater improvements on a variety of indices of marital adjustment compared to controls, and the BMT groups also enjoyed a greater degree of sobriety over a short-term follow-up. Two other studies found a "cross over" effect in which patients who received BMT began to have better drinking outcomes than those who did not after the first year of follow-up (McCrady et al., 1986; Stout, McCrady, Longabaugh, Noel, & Beattie, 1989). Studies also have indicated that patients in conjoint therapy are less likely to drop out of treatment (Noel, McCrady, Stout, & Fisher-Nelson, 1987), and that therapy aimed at improving the marriage as a whole (e.g., BMT) seems to work better than couples therapy focused strictly on alcohol-related problems (McCrady, 1986).

There is also evidence that BMT can be effective as an aftercare intervention. O'Farrell and colleagues found that a version of BMT that included relapse prevention techniques (Marlatt & Gordon, 1985) and was delivered as an aftercare intervention led to better drinking outcomes for the alcoholics than did a no aftercare control condition (O'Farrell, Choquette, Cutter, Brown, & McCourt, in press).

## BRIEF INTERVENTIONS

In recent years there has been increased interest in alternative treatment options for different subpopulations of individuals with alcohol problems and for those who are at risk for such problems. "Brief" interventions, which are aimed at individuals who are "early career" problem drinkers, have been among the more intensively studied of these alternative approaches. This work received considerable mention in the Institute of Medicine (1990) report on alcohol treatment. In this section we summarize the clinical research that has been completed on brief interventions. Our comments draw heavily from two excellent, recent reviews of the topic (Babor, 1992; Bien, Miller, & Tonigan, 1992).

*Definition.* Before summarizing the results of the research, it is important to define what makes an intervention "brief." Not surprisingly, what is considered brief is relative to what the comparison is, so there is no absolute standard. However, the major features of such interventions, as they have been implemented in clinical research, can be described. These features were outlined by Babor (1992), as follows. First, brief interventions have been targeted to individuals with less severe dependence on alcohol and less severe alcohol-related problems. Second, brief interventions have lasted from 1-3 sessions, each of which generally has been 5-30 minutes long. The content of these sessions has varied across studies. Third, the goals of brief interventions have included abstinence from alcohol and, because such interventions have not been used with severely dependent individuals, moderate, nonproblem drinking. Brief interventions also may include goals of improved general health and social functioning. Finally, the settings where brief interventions have been implemented have covered a range, from primary health care settings, to outpatient community mental health settings, to work settings. These four sets of factors, in combination, result in a variety of interventions and contexts in the study of what has been called brief interventions.

*Outcomes of Brief Interventions.* Controlled clinical trials of brief interventions date back to the 1960s and across a span of 14 countries. From the Babor (1992) and Bien et al. (1992) reviews of this research, the conclusions are consistent. First, brief interventions typically are more effective (in terms of alcohol use, general health, or social functioning) than no intervention. Another result is that brief interventions also often have comparable effects to those of traditional, more intense and longer-term programs. Furthermore, brief interventions have been shown to increase the effectiveness of later treatment. These results have been surprising to many, and have significant implications for the delivery of alcohol treatment. In addition, the consistency of these findings across such diverse settings and intervention parameters lends confidence that brief interventions have real effects.

## COST EFFECTIVENESS OF ALCOHOLISM TREATMENTS

Studies have consistently shown that treatment for newly identified alcoholics is cost effective. That is, the reductions in total health care costs following treatment are greater than the costs of the treatment itself (Holder, 1987; Saxe, Dougherty, Esty, & Fine, 1983). The more expensive treatments for alcoholism may not be the most cost effective, however. In a recent review article, Holder et al. (1991) examined the effectiveness, benefits to society, and costs of 21 different approaches to alcoholism treatments. Over 200 controlled studies were included in the review. These authors found that the relationship between treatment costs and treatment effectiveness was negative; that is, the more expensive the treatment, the less evidence there was of its effectiveness.

One of the limitations of this review is that not enough controlled studies of two of the most popular alcoholism treatments, AA and 28-day residential programs, had been done to evaluate their cost effectiveness. However, the costs associated with these two interventions were partially examined in the Walsh et al. (1991) study described earlier. Although the costs were initially lower in the AA only condition, a higher percentage of patients in this condition required hospitalization at some point in the follow-up. When the costs stemming from initial inpatient treatment as well as any additional inpatient treatments during the two year follow-up were tallied, costs for patients referred to AA without inpatient treatment were only 10% less than costs for those in the inpatient condition.

## PATIENT-TREATMENT MATCHING

Although some treatments for alcoholism appear to be more effective than others, no one intervention has emerged as clearly superior. There is, however, a fair amount of evidence to suggest that certain kinds of patients do better in specific treatment modalities. A number of studies have found that patients with either less social support or stability, a greater degree of alcohol dependence or problem severity, or some degree of psychiatric comorbidity seem to benefit more from inpatient treatment (McLellan et al., 1983; Miller & Hester, 1986b; Nace, 1989; Orford, Oppenheimer, & Edwards, 1976). Clearly, alcoholic patients who are also engaging in extremely self-destructive behavior, acutely suicidal, or violent may require inpatient care (Miller, 1989; Nace, 1989).

Patient-treatment matches involving psychiatric comorbidity were also identified in a study of aftercare treatment (Kadden et al., 1989; Cooney et al., 1991). Patients with higher global psychopathology ratings or higher sociopathy scores had better drinking outcomes in cognitive-behavioral group aftercare than in interactional group aftercare. On the other hand, those with neuropsychological impairments did better in the interactional group treatment.

However, cognitive-behavioral mood management training was not as effective for patients with higher levels of anxiety or stronger urges to drink during treatment in a study by Rohsenow et al. (1991). In this study, communication skills training benefited a broader range of patients, regardless of education, anxiety, or urges to drink.

A number of personality variables have emerged as potential matching variables. Patients with a low "conceptual level"–those with a preference for simpler rules, fewer abstract cognitive constructs, and greater dependence on authority–do better with more directive and structured treatments while the opposite is true for those with high conceptual level (McLachlan, 1972; 1974). Patients with low self-esteem appear to do particularly badly in confrontational groups (Annis & Chan, 1983). Functioning in the families of alcoholic patients with low levels of autonomy improves to a greater degree when the alcoholics are treated *without* other family members, whereas with high autonomy alcoholics, family functioning improves more when other family members are included in the treatment (McKay, Longabaugh, Beattie, Maisto, & Noel, in press b). Finally, Miller (1992) reported that alcohol abusers who believed alcoholism was a bad habit did better in behavioral treatment, whereas those who believed it was a disease did better in 12-Step oriented treatment.

There is also evidence that patients' degree of social support can act as a matching variable in outpatient treatment. In a study of the Community Reinforcement Approach (CRA), single patients did much better in the full CRA condition, whereas married patients did as well when they only received Antabuse. In a study comparing social-learning based conjoint and nonconjoint outpatient alcoholism treatments (Longabaugh, Beattie, Noel, Stout, & Malloy, in press), patients who did not receive support for their sobriety from family and friends did particularly badly if they were in the conjoint condition. These findings highlight the complexity of appropriate patient-treatment matching. Not only do the characteristics of the person and treatment need to be considered, but also those of the person's posttreatment environment.

Finally, another approach that has been taken to match patients to treatments involves the specific timing of interventions and the concept of a continuum of care. In this approach, patients' treatment needs are thought to change over time in a predictable fashion. Matching involves delivering the proper intervention at the appropriate time. Two comprehensive, medical model-based systems that have been developed, the Cleveland Admission, Discharge, and Transfer Criteria (Hoffman, Halikas, & Mee-Lee, 1987) and the American Society of Addiction Medicine Placement Criteria (1990), call for matching patients to treatments on the basis of problem or symptom severity in a number of areas. In both systems, guidelines for placing patients in treatments of different intensities, ranging from self-help programs all the way to hospital-based inpatient programs, are spelled out in detail. With the Cleveland Criteria, for example, patients are rated on seven dimensions: withdrawal severity, physical complications, psychiatric complications, life areas impairments, treatment acceptance, loss of control, and recovery environment. Greater problem severity in any area calls for more intensive and/or restrictive treatment. As problem severity drops, patients advance to less intensive forms of treatment. Therefore, these criteria provide comprehensive guidelines for initial treatment placement and for continuum of care.

Despite the obvious appeal of such an approach to patient-treatment matching, initial research findings suggest that these comprehensive guidelines to treatment placement may require further development before they are valid. McKay, McLellan, and Alterman (1992) found that many alcoholic patients treated in a day hospital rehabilitation program met one or more of the Cleveland Criteria for inpatient rehabilitation. These patients were therefore "mismatched" to day hospital, according to the criteria. However, when these patients were compared to those properly matched to day hospital on a number of outcome measures, including treatment completion, posttreatment drinking frequency and severity, and psychosocial problem severity, there were no differences between the two groups.

Prochaska, DiClemente, and colleagues also have asserted that the timing of interventions is important. However, their matching system is based on a psychological construct, readiness to change, rather than symptom severity. According to the theory, the behavior change process consists of five stages: precontemplation, contemplation, preparation, action, and maintenance (Prochaska & Di-Clemente, 1992). The likelihood that individuals will stop their alcoholic behavior in the near future is seen as a function of their current stage of change. For example, alcoholics at the precontemplation stage may benefit to a greater degree from interventions designed to move them to the next stage, rather than from an intensive treatment intervention that they likely would resist. There is some preliminary evidence that correctly matching treatment interventions to an individual's stage of change improves treatment outcome (Prochaska, DiClemente, & Norcross, 1992).

## TREATMENT PROCESS

Another approach to improving the efficacy of alcoholism treatment has been to identify treatment-related factors, such as goals and processes, that are associated with better outcomes. These studies are usually naturalistic and correlational, rather than experimental, which means that it is not possible to determine whether the process measures are actually exerting a causal influence on outcome. However, the identification of processes and goals that predict outcome does generate hypotheses concerning the "active ingredients" of treatment. These hypotheses can be used to develop new therapeutic interventions or modify existing ones.

One of the central goals of alcoholism treatment is to increase the alcoholic's ability to cope with various potentially stressful internal states and/or external situations without relapsing. Two aspects of coping have been studied empirically: alcoholics' beliefs concerning their coping abilities (i.e., self-efficacy) and the type of coping responses they typically employ. Self-efficacy essentially is the belief that one will be able to cope successfully with potentially problematic situations (Bandura, 1977). In several studies, increases in self-efficacy or higher self-efficacy at the end of alcoholism treatment predicted better drinking outcomes during follow-up (Burling, Reilly, Moltzen, & Ziff, 1989; McKay, Maisto, & O'Farrell, in press c). In studies of coping responses, the strategies alcoholics use to cope with high risk situations have been divided into active versus avoidant approaches. Active coping refers to cognitive or behavioral strategies aimed at problem solving or mastery, whereas avoidant coping refers to staying away from the high risk situation. Alcoholics who report more frequent use of active coping typically have better drinking outcomes than those who rely to a greater degree on avoidance (Edwards et al., 1987; Moos et al., 1990).

A number of other treatment goals or processes have been studied empirically. There is evidence that greater commitment to abstinence at the end of treatment predicts better short-term drinking outcomes (Hall, Havassy, & Wasserman, 1990). For alcoholics low in autonomy, improvements in family functioning during treatment predicted better posttreatment drinking outcomes (McKay, Longabaugh, Beattie, Maisto, & Noel, in press d). In high autonomy alcoholics, however, changes in family functioning were unrelated to drinking outcomes, presumably because these individuals are less affected by the state of their social relations. Finally, longer stays in treatment and treatment completion have predicted better drinking outcomes, even after various pretreatment characteristics of alcoholics have been controlled for (McKay et al., in press a; Moos et al., 1990).

## *RELAPSE PREVENTION*

In the last decade, there has been increasing interest in the "maintenance phase" of recovery, the period that follows the end of initial or primary treatment (Brownell, Marlatt, Lichtenstein, & Wilson, 1986). During this period, alcoholics either are able to maintain the gains they achieved in treatment (e.g., abstinence or controlled drinking), or they experience a resumption of problematic drinking (i.e., relapses). The determinants and predictors of relapse have been extensively studied by Marlatt and colleagues, and by other investigators. Retrospective reports by alcoholics suggest that relapses tend to occur in certain situations, including unpleasant emotional states, interpersonal conflicts, and pleasant social gathering such as parties (Maisto, O'Farrell, Connors, McKay, & Pelcovits, 1988; Marlatt & Gordon, 1985).

Studies of the determinants of relapse have led to the development of relapse prevention interventions that are designed to equip alcoholics to cope successfully with high stress situations after primary rehabilitation has ended (Annis & Davis, 1989; Marlatt & Gordon, 1985). These interventions are typically based on social-learning theory and involve techniques from cognitive-behavior therapy, including detailed assessments of cues and vulnerabilities for relapse, interventions to increase coping skills and self-efficacy, and the use of role playing, rehearsal, and homework assignments.

One of the more systematic approaches to relapse prevention has been developed by Annis and Davis (1989). This approach is based on self-efficacy theory (Bandura, 1977) and makes use of standardized assessment instruments to identify areas of relapse vulnerability. At first, interventions are directed primarily at helping patients avoid risky situations. After this initial phase, interventions are focused on improving coping abilities and increasing mastery and self-efficacy in situations of relatively low risk. This is primarily accomplished through homework assignments, completed between sessions, that involve practicing the appropriate coping response while exposed to the situation. After the alcoholic has experienced some success in coping with less risky situations without relapsing, the same process is undertaken with increasingly risky situations.

The research that has been done with relapse prevention interventions indicates that this approach generally does not lead to better results than other types of aftercare interventions (Annis & Davis, 1988; Kadden et al., 1989). However, there is evidence from these studies that alcoholics who can specify under what situations they usually drink and those with higher psychopathology or sociopathy scores do better if they receive relapse prevention rather than more traditional forms of aftercare.

## EFFECTIVENESS OF SELF-HELP GROUPS

Many alcoholism treatment programs are based to some degree on the principals of Alcoholics Anonymous (AA), and greater involvement with self-help groups during and after treatment is widely thought to lead to better drinking outcomes (McCrady & Irvine, 1989; Vaillant, 1983). Furthermore, anecdotal reports given by clinicians and AA members about the effectiveness of AA suggest that those who get involved with AA have a better chance at recovery. However, the effectiveness of AA has not been evaluated in any randomized studies due to a host of ethical and practical problems associated with attempting to assign alcoholics to not go to AA (McCrady & Irvine, 1989; McKay et al., 1991; Miller & Hester, 1986). Most studies of AA therefore have had to rely on correlational designs.

First, a number of studies have examined the relationship between degree of participation in AA and drinking outcomes. Moos and colleagues (1990) found small but significant relationships between more frequent attendance at AA during and after rehabilitation and better drinking outcomes, after patient characteristics were controlled for. Vaillant (1983) reported that AA was only effective for alcoholic men who attended meetings frequently over a prolonged period of time. In a recent study of alcoholic day hospital patients, greater participation in AA at three months posttreatment predicted better drinking outcomes three months later, even after degree of success in day hospital was controlled for (McKay et al., in press a). Second, a number of patient characteristics appear to predict involvement in AA. There is some evidence that patients with greater severity of drinking problems, affective rather than cognitive focus, a concern about purpose and meaning in life, better interpersonal skills, and a high need for affiliation are good candidates for AA (Emrick, 1987; McCrady & Irvine, 1989).

## TREATMENT OF DUAL-DIAGNOSIS ALCOHOLICS

Treatment of the "dual diagnosed" patient has been discussed in the clinical literature for many years but has received wide-spread research attention only in the last decade. The term dual diagnosis–other common terms are co-morbidity and dual disorder–refers here to a diagnosis of a substance use disorder and at least one other disorder. In DSM-III-R terms, that other disorder may be an Axis 1 or Axis 2 disorder.

The interest in dual diagnosis patients stems from their prevalence in both nonclinical and clinical settings. For example, the Epidemiological Catchment Area (ECA) study was conducted in the early 1980s and involved personal and telephone interviews of 20,000 people in five major U.S. cities who lived in households, group homes, and long-term institutions. From this data base Helzer and Pryzbeck (1988) reported that among men with a DSM-III lifetime diagnosis of alcohol abuse or dependence, 19% had a lifetime diagnosis of other drug abuse or dependence, 15% antisocial personality disorder, and 13% phobic disorder. The rates for the total population of men, in contrast, were 7%, 4%, and 9%, respectively. This discrepancy in rates of diagnoses among alcohol diagnosed women and the total population of women was similar to that in men. A national survey of psychiatric and substance use disorders in the general population was recently completed by the University of Michigan, and the preliminary findings of that study confirm and add to the ECA study findings (Kessler, 1992).

Directly relevant to this article is the high rate of other Axis 1 or Axis 2 disorders among individuals who present for alcohol or other drug treatment (Group for the Advancement of Psychiatry, 1991). In this regard, Kosten and Kleber (1988) noted dual diagnosis patients constitute as many as 80% of identified substance abusers. The diagnoses that seem to co-occur most often with the substance use disorders are affective and anxiety disorders, psychotic disorders, and antisocial personality disorder (Kosten & Kleber, 1988; Rounsaville, Dolinsky, Babor, & Meyer, 1987).

*Dual Diagnosis and Alcohol (and Other Drug) Treatment.* Besides prevalence, the subject of dual diagnosis is occupying so much clinical and research attention because co-occurring psychiatric diagnosis and psychiatric problem severity predict treatment outcome. Table 1 presents a sample of more recent studies of the relationship between psychiatric severity or diagnosis co-occurring with alcohol or drug use disorder. As Table 1 shows, the studies cover a diversity of patient populations and treatment settings. The predominant finding in this work has been that either the presence of a co-occurring psychiatric disorder or a greater degree of psychiatric symptom severity predicts poorer alcohol and drug treatment outcomes. This finding holds for outcome criteria of substance use and other areas of functioning, such as social functioning and psychological functioning.

The research also provides information concerning matching the content of alcohol and drug treatment to the patient's psychiatric status, although the research base is much scarcer than that regarding prediction of treatment outcome. It appears, essentially, that

TABLE 1. Psychiatric Functioning and Outcome of Alcohol and Drug Treatment

| Authors (Year) | Patients | Settings |
|---|---|---|
| Glenn & Parsons (1991) | Men and women who met criteria for "alcoholism," rated on depressive symptoms | Community alcoholism treatment centers |
| Kosten et al. (1989) | Men and women opiate addicts assessed for DSM-III Axis 2 disorder | Inpatient and outpatient substance abuse treatment settings |
| McClellan (1986) (summary of several studies published elsewhere) | Male veterans, alcohol or other drug abusers and rated on Addiction Severity Index psychiatric severity | Inpatient and outpatient alcohol and drug treatment programs |
| Ojehegan et al. (1990) | Men and women DSM-III alcohol abuse or dependent, rated on psychiatric diagnosis and symptoms | Alcohol outpatient program |
| Powell et al. (1992) | Men, alcohol dependent, and one additional psychiatric syndrome | Inpatient alcohol treatment program |
| Rounsaville & Kleber (1986) (summary of several studies published elsewhere) | Men and women opiate addicts and rated on psychiatric diagnosis and psychiatric severity | Patients presented for assignment to inpatient or outpatient drug treatment programs |

patients who have psychiatric problems may show improved outcomes if psychotherapy is part of their alcohol and drug treatment. The empirical base of this idea consists primarily of one controlled clinical trial that was conducted by McClellan and his colleagues and published initially in the early 1980s (see McClellan, 1986).

Fortunately, this important finding generated a substantial amount of research interest in patient X treatment matching, the most important example of which is a national multisite matching controlled clinical trial (Project MATCH) funded by the National Institute on Alcohol Abuse and Alcoholism that is in progress. Patient psychiatric diagnosis and psychiatric status is one set of matching variables that will be analyzed in Project MATCH.

*Model of Care of the Dual Diagnosed Patient.* Traditionally, the dual diagnosed patient has "fallen through the cracks" of the treatment system. That is, these patients did not fit in the standard defined provinces of either the substance abuse or mental health care systems (Minkoff, 1991). This problem continues and has generated discussion of models of care of the dual diagnosed patient. Two major models are the hybrid or integrated model, and the parallel or sequential model. The hybrid model implies that the dual diagnosed patient receives care for both types of problems at the same time and in one treatment setting. In the parallel model, services may be delivered concurrently or serially in different treatment settings (Ridgely, 1991).

The advantages of the hybrid system are the system's efficiency and consistency of care. A practical problem in implementing the model, however, results from differences among dual diagnosed patients in the nature of their problems and in their degree of motivation for treatment. As a result, it is questionable that enough hybrid programs could be developed to meet the diversity of dual diagnosed patients. A major advantage of the parallel system is the flexibility it affords the case manager in planning services for the different types of problems. For example, individuals may be more motivated to agree to intense treatment for their psychiatric problems than for their substance use problems. Treatment for the latter may have to be less intense in order to engage the patient in any treatment at all. The major disadvantage of the parallel model is the great burden that is placed in case managers to maintain treatment continuity through multiple episodes of treatment in different care systems.

Both the hybrid and parallel models of care are already in practice in the United States. Unfortunately, there are no systematic data on what the more effective model of care is. Therefore, this is a pressing research question. Furthermore, there are many patient and treatment system characteristics that can be the bases of matching prescriptions. One such matching variable might be patient motivation to change a particular problem behavior. One prominent model of change that has generated considerable interest in the addictions area in Prochaska and DiClemente's (1992) stages of change model. A similar model of change was developed independently in work with dual diagnosed patients by Osher and Kofoed (1989). It seems that such models could be applied productively to investigate patient motivation to change a problem behavior and selection of a model of care.

## PHARMACOTHERAPY

In this section, we review evidence concerning the effectiveness of disulfiram (Antabuse), a medication that is used to deter alcoholics from drinking by producing an aversive reaction after alcohol is ingested. We will also discuss recent findings that suggest that certain drugs may act as anti-craving agents with alcoholics. The use of psychotropic medications with alcoholics will be addressed in the Discussion section.

Most controlled studies have demonstrated that the benefit obtained by disulfiram therapy is accounted for by a placebo effect rather than the drug itself. However, several studies concluded that a certain subset of patients are more likely to benefit from disulfiram than from placebo or no treatment. In a large, VA multi-center study (Fuller et al., 1986), older and more socially stable men who relapsed during the follow-up had fewer drinking days if they were in the treatment condition receiving a therapeutic dose of disulfiram. These results replicated an earlier study (Baekeland, Lundwall, Kissin, & Shanahan, 1971) in which middle-aged men with the following characteristics were more likely to benefit from disulfiram: greater social stability; a longer history of heavy drinking; a history of delirium tremens; good motivation, as manifested by contact with AA and/or abstinence at intake; and not being treated with antidepressant medication. According to Fuller, "the middle-aged alcoholic who has relapsed, has some degree of social stability, and is not significantly depressed is the most suitable candidate for disulfiram therapy" (1989, p. 119). Furthermore, the side effects of disulfiram and potential danger of disulfiram-ethanol reaction contraindicate its use in patients with a wide array of medical and psychiatric conditions and in pregnant women (Fuller, 1989).

There is also strong evidence for the effectiveness of disulfiram in preventing relapse when it is used in a comprehensive behavior therapy treatment program. In several such programs, a contract was drawn up which specified that disulfiram ingestion was to be monitored by a significant other (Azrin et al., 1982; O'Farrell et al., 1985). Since compliance is a major obstacle to the effectiveness of disulfiram treatment, this sort of behavioral contracting may be an important component of the treatment.

Pharmacotherapy may also prove to be useful in decreasing alcoholics' craving for alcohol. A recent randomized study found that naltrexone, an opiate receptor blocker, significantly decreased self-reported craving levels in alcoholics when used as an adjunct to psychosocial treatment (Volpicelli, Alterman, Hayashida, & O'Brien, 1992). Furthermore, alcoholics who received naltrexone were less likely to progress to a full-blown relapse if they did drink, compared to those who did not receive naltrexone.

## DISCUSSION

The research reviewed in this article indicates that there are many exciting developments in the treatment of alcohol use disorders. In this section, we will briefly summarize the more important findings, identify several under-studied and/or unresolved issues, and offer suggestions for further research.

*Patient-Treatment Matching.* There is increasingly compelling evidence that (a) no one treatment is superior with all alcoholics, and (b) proper matching of alcoholics to appropriate treatments produces better outcomes. We now have some empirical evidence to indicate which alcoholics will benefit to a greater degree from inpatient, cognitive-behavioral, interactional, and conjoint interventions. Project MATCH, referred to earlier, will generate considerably more information on which alcoholics do better in 12-step focused, cognitive-behavioral, and brief intervention treatments. Matching alcoholics to a continuum of care on the basis of their symptom severity and/or readiness to change also appears to have promise, although there is less empirical evidence for this. It would be worthwhile, for example, to determine whether a brief inpatient stay (e.g., 2-4 days) followed by outpatient rehabilitation would lead to higher treatment completion rates and better drinking outcomes than outpatient treatment alone.

*Treatment Process.* Research on treatment process has identified several variables, such as the use of active coping responses, high self-efficacy, commitment to abstinence, and treatment completion, which predict better drinking outcomes. However, little is known about the specific "active ingredients" that bring about changes in these behaviors and beliefs or otherwise produce better drinking outcomes. For example, although most rehabilitation programs make extensive use of didactic sessions, there is very little evidence that these sessions are associated with better outcomes (Miller & Hester, 1986b; Moos et al., 1990). More research is needed to identify the specific treatment processes, components, and goals that facilitate recovery. Such investigations should also consider the possibility that different processes are important at different points in recovery. For example, certain goals or processes during primary treatment may be important because they facilitate continued participation in aftercare or posttreatment self-help groups, which in turn can promote long-term abstinence (McKay et al., in press a).

*Brief Interventions.* Studies have shown that brief interventions can be effective in reducing drinking. Furthermore, they are highly cost effective (Holder et al., 1991). At the same time, the research on brief interventions has generated a number of questions. First, what combination of parameters might be most efficient and effective in delivering brief intervention? Variables to consider in this regard include session content, duration, number, and spacing (if there is more than one session). In conjunction with this question is the issue of the relative effectiveness of different brief interventions. Furthermore, if brief interventions behave as do more traditional alcohol treatment protocols and settings, there is the central question of matching patient characteristics to brief intervention and setting characteristics. As Bien et al. (1992) noted, in research to date on brief intervention, subject populations have been relatively homogeneous. However, there are patient characteristics that may have major significance for matching to brief interventions and thus warrant systematic research. Examples include patient motivation to change patterns of alcohol use, degree of severity of alcohol dependence and problems, and presence of dual diagnoses.

Finally, a core question concerns why brief interventions work at all. Bien et al. (1992) provided a stimulating discussion of the elements that they viewed as common to the brief interventions that have been studied; two or more of the elements were present in each of the studies these authors reviewed. The six elements were summarized by the acronym FRAMES: *F*eedback of personal risk or impairment; Emphasis on Personal *R*esponsibility for change; clear *A*dvice to change; providing a *M*enu of alternative strategies for behavior change; therapeutic *E*mpathy as a counseling style; and enhancement of client *S*elf-Efficacy, or optimism. These elements can serve as hypotheses about the process of brief interventions. Important questions are which elements may be necessary for change to occur, what combinations of elements are important for different patient populations, and the degree of presence of an element that is required in order to achieve an effect.

*Dual-Diagnosis Patients.* The research on treatment of dual diagnosis patients has also raised important questions. First, there is a fundamental need for longitudinal studies of individuals with co-occurring substance use and other psychiatric disorders. Drake, McLaughlin, Pepper, and Minkoff (1991) noted the lack of information on reasons for substance use among dual disordered patients. They also noted the lack of good empirical information on the development and maintenance of substance use patterns, and their interaction with psychiatric symptoms.

One reason for conducting longitudinal research on dual diagnosis patients is that the resulting data will be extremely valuable in furthering the conceptual and theoretical development of the field. For example, a widespread assumption among clinicians and researchers alike is that dual diagnosis patients use alcohol or other drugs to "self-medicate"–to assuage or ease their psychiatric distress (e.g., Khantzian, 1985). However, there is little empirical information to support such broad applicability of this hypothesis, and some data that are not consistent with it (e.g., Galanter, Castaneda, & Ferman, 1988; Weiss & Mirin, 1987). Longitudinal data would not only help to further theoretical advances about substance use in individuals with psychiatric problems, but also would give a better understanding of the functions (Haynes & O'Brien, 1990) in general of alcohol and other drugs among these individuals. Related to this point, Bachrach (1986-1987) commented that psychiatric patients are a heterogeneous group who have a range of determinants and consequences of substance use.

Longitudinal research also would lend information to a vital question for practitioners who work with dual diagnosis patients: which is the "primary" diagnosis? Schuckit (1985) has written extensively on this question. He defined primary and secondary by temporal order of symptom appearance. If symptoms of psychiatric difficulties precede any evidence of problems with alcohol or other drugs, then psychiatric problems are primary. If the reverse is true, then the substance use disorder is primary. Psychiatric symptoms that are primary may persist after detoxification and lead to an increased risk for relapse.

This suggests that the use of psychotropic medications may be central to the management of certain psychiatric disorders. Although there may be different degrees of agreement with this statement, dependent on the disorder in question, mental health treatment providers tend to be open to the use of psychotropic medications in treatment of their patients. However, this is not the case when treating the dual diagnosed patient. The controversy revolves around several major questions. First, there are philosophical differences among treatment providers, especially those who identify most closely with treatment of substance abusers, about the use of drugs (psychotropic medications) in the treatment of individuals who have problems with alcohol or other drugs. A second major question is the abuse potential of the medication: How likely is the medication to become a drug of abuse rather than a drug of treatment? Most notorious in this regard is the benzodiazepine family of drugs. Finally, there is the question of the pharmacological interaction of the psychotropic medication with alcohol and other drugs. Primary here is the potential for using both the prescribed and nonprescribed drugs in sufficient quantities to increase the chances of intentional or inadvertent suicide (Drake et al., 1991; Minkoff, 1991).

These important questions have received much clinical attention, but extremely limited systematic research. Some basic items for a research agenda on this topic are as follows. In treating individuals who present for alcohol or drug treatment, does prescription of psychotropic medications to modify psychiatric symptoms enhance outcomes, compared to using nondrug treatments? Second, who are the best candidates for medication use? A third fundamental question is what is the frequency and pattern of compliance with and abuse of prescription of psychotropic medications among substance abusers who are given such treatment? Finally, are psychotropic medications that have low abuse potential effective adjuncts to psychosocial treatments (e.g., Malcom, Anton, Randall, Johnston, Brady, and Theros, 1992)?

*Social Supports.* One of the more persuasive findings in the literature reviewed here concerns the importance of social support to the recovery process, both during and after treatment. Higher levels of family dysfunction at intake and at follow-up have been associated with worse drinking outcomes (McKay, Longabaugh, Beattie, Maisto, & Noel, 1992; Moos & Moos, 1984), and increases in family dysfunction during treatment have predicted poorer outcomes for lower autonomy alcoholics (McKay et al., in press d). Furthermore, behavioral marital therapy generally appears to be a highly effective form of treatment (Holder et al., 1991). Participation in self-help groups, which often provides considerable social support, has also been associated with the maintenance of abstinence following treatment (Vaillant, 1983). However, the social environment can also be problematic. There is evidence that patients who are treated with significant others who are not supportive of abstinence have particularly bad drinking outcomes (Longabaugh et al., in press). Additional research is needed to determine which individuals profit from what type of social support and how to better facilitate the process of linking alcoholics to forms of social support that are conducive to maintaining alcohol and drug-free living.

*Increased Emphasis on Life-Style Enhancement.* Finally, Vaillant (1983) and various clinical theorists have observed that alcoholics who are able to maintain long term abstinence often become highly invested in and devote considerable amounts of their time to something other than alcohol. For some alcoholics, this involves participation in 12-Step programs, religious beliefs, helping others, or supporting certain causes. Others make major life changes, such as going to school, changing careers, developing new hobbies or skills, becoming physically active, or beginning new relationships. These activities all increase self-esteem, take up free time that might otherwise be problematic, and provide powerful incentives to remain abstinent. Most alcoholism treatments, regardless of their setting or orientation, are primarily focused on helping individuals to cope with various stressors without resorting to the use of alcohol. It may also be useful to devote more research efforts to devising treatment protocols aimed at facilitating patients' efforts to discover and nurture their interests and passions as well as their efforts to develop activities that are enjoyable and health-enhancing.

## REFERENCES

Annis, H.M., & Chan, D. (1983). The differential treatment model: Empirical evidence from a personality typology of adult offenders. *Criminal Justice and Behavior, 10,* 159-173.

Annis, H.M., & Davis, C.S. (1989). Relapse prevention. In R.K. Hester & W.R. Miller (Eds.), *Handbook of alcoholism treatment approaches* (pp. 170-182). New York: Pergamon Press.

American Society of Addiction Medicine (1990). *Patient placement criteria for the treatment of psychoactive substance use disorders.*

Azrin, N.H. (1976). Improvements in the community reinforcement approach to alcoholism. *Behavior Research and Therapy, 14,* 339-348.

Azrin, N.H., Sisson, R.W., Meyers, R., & Godley, M. (1982). A social-systems approach to resocializing alcoholics in the community. *Journal of Studies on Alcohol, 43,* 1115-1123.

Babor, T.F. (1992). *Avoiding the horrible and beastly sin of drunkenness: Does dissuasion make a difference?* Unpublished manuscript, University of Connecticut School of Medicine.

Bachrach, L. (1986-1987). The content of care for the chronic mental patient with substance abuse problems. *Psychiatric Quarterly, 58,* 3-14.

Baekeland, F., Lundwall, L., Kissin, B., & Shanahan, T. (1971). Correlates of outcome in disulfiram treatment. *Journal of Nervous and Mental Disease, 153,* 1-9.

Bandura, A. (1977). Self efficacy: Toward a unifying theory of behavioral change. *Psychological Review, 84,* 191-215.

Bien, T.H., Miller, W.R., & Tonigan J.S. (1992). *Brief interventions for alcohol problems: A review.* Unpublished manuscript, Department of Psychology, University of New Mexico.

Brownell, K.D., Marlatt, G.A., Lichtenstein, E., & Wilson, G.T. (1986). Understanding and preventing relapse. *American Psychologist, 41,* 765-782.

Burling, T.A., Reilly, P.M., Moltzen, J.O., & Ziff, D.C. (1989). Self-efficacy and relapse among inpatient drug and alcohol abusers: A predictor of outcome. *Journal of Studies on Alcohol, 50,* 354-360.

Chaney, E.F. (1989). Social skills training. In R.K. Hester & W.R. Miller (Eds.), *Handbook of alcoholism treatment approaches* (pp. 206-221). New York: Pergamon Press.

Cooney, N.L., Kadden, R.M., Litt, M.D., & Getter, H. (1991). Matching alcoholics to coping skills or interactional therapies: Two-year follow-up results. *Journal of Consulting and Clinical Psychology, 59,* 598-601.

Drake, R.E., McLaughlin, P., Pepper, B., & Minkoff, K. (1991). Dual diagnosis of major mental illness and substance disorder: An overview. In K. Minkoff & R.E. Drake (Eds.), *Dual diagnosis of major mental illness and substance disorder* (pp. 3-12). San Francisco: Jossey-Bass, Inc.

Edwards, G., Brown, D., Duckitt, A. et al. (1987). Outcome of alcoholism: The structure of patient attributions as to what causes change. *British Journal of Addictions, 82,* 533-545.

Emrick, C. (1987). Alcoholics Anonymous: Affiliation processes and effectiveness as treatment. *Alcoholism: Clinical and Experimental Research, 11,* 416-423.

Fuller, R.K. (1989). Antidipsotropic medications. In R.K. Hester & W.R. Miller (Eds.), *Handbook of alcoholism treatment approaches* (pp. 117-127). New York: Pergamon Press.

Fuller, R.K., Branchey, L., Brightwell, D.R., Derman, R.M., Emrick, C.D., Iber, F.L., James, K.E., Lacoursiere, R.B., Lee, K.K., Lowenstam, I., Maany, I., Neiderheiser, D., Nocks, J.J., & Shaw, S. (1986). Disulfiram treatment of alcoholism: A Veterans Administration cooperative study. *Journal of Nervous and Mental Disease, 256,* 449-1455.

Galanter, M., Castaneda, R., & Freeman, J. (1989). Substance abuse among general psychiatric patients: Place of presentation, diagnosis, and treatment. *American Journal of Drug and Alcohol Abuse, 14,* 211-235.

Glenn, S.W., & Parsons, O.A. (1991). Prediction of resumption of drinking in post treatment alcoholics. *The International Journal of the Addictions, 26,* 237-254.

Group for the Advancement of Psychiatry (1991). Substance abuse disorders: A psychiatric priority. *American Journal of Psychiatry, 148,* 1291-1300.

Hall S.M., Havassy B.E., & Wasserman D.A. (1990). Commitment to abstinence and acute stress in relapse to alcohol, opiates, and nicotine. *Journal of Consulting and Clinical Psychology, 58,* 175-181.

Havassy, B.E., Hall, S.M., & Wasserman, D.A. (in press). Social support and relapse: Commonalities among alcoholics, opiate users, and cigarette smokers. *Addictive Behaviors.*

Haynes, S.N., & O'Brien, W.H. (1990). Functional analysis in behavior therapy. *Clinical Psychology Review, 10*, 649-668.

Helzer, J.E., & Pryzbeck, T.R. (1988). The co-occurrence of alcoholism with other psychiatric disorders in the general population and its impact on treatment. *Journal of Studies on Alcohol, 49*, 219-224.

Hoffman, N.G., Halikas, J.A., & Mee-Lee, D. (1987). The *Cleveland Admission, Discharge, and Transfer Criteria: Model for chemical dependency treatment programs.* Cleveland, Northern Ohio Chemical Dependency Treatment Directors Association.

Holder, H.D. (1987). Alcoholism treatment and potential health care cost saving. *Medical Care, 25*, 52-71.

Holder, H.D., Longabaugh, R., Miller, W.R., & Rubonis, A.V. (1991). The cost effectiveness of treatment for alcohol problems: A first approximation. *Journal of Studies on Alcohol, 52*, 517-540.

Hunt, G.M., & Azrin, N.H. (1973). A community reinforcement approach to alcoholism. *Behavior Research and Therapy, 11*, 91-104.

Institute of Medicine (1990). *Prevention and treatment of alcohol problems: Research opportunities.* Washington, D.C.: National Academy Press.

Kadden, R.M., Cooney, N.L., Getter, H., & Litt, M.D. (1989). Matching alcoholics to coping skills or interactional therapies: Post-treatment results. *Journal of Consulting and Clinical Psychology, 57*(6), 698-704.

Kessler, R. (1992). *The National Comorbidity Survey: Introduction and overview.* Paper presented at the NIMH/NIAAA Workshop on Advances in Research on Co-occurring Disorders, Bethesda, MD, April 30-May 1.

Khantzian, E.J. (1985). The self-medication hypothesis of addictive disorders: Focus on heroin and cocaine dependence. *The American Journal of Psychiatry, 142*, 1259-1264.

Kosten, T.R., & Kleber, H.D. (1988). Differential diagnosis of psychiatric comorbidity in substance abusers. *Journal of Substance Abuse Treatment, 5*, 201-206.

Kosten, T.A., Kosten, T.R., & Rounsaville, B.J. (1989). Personality disorders in opiate addicts show prognostic specificity. *Journal of Substance Abuse Treatment, 6*, 163-168.

Longabaugh, R. (1988). Longitudinal outcome studies. In R.M. Rose & J. Barrett (Eds.), *Alcoholism: Origins and outcome.* New York: Raven Press, Ltd, pp. 267-280.

Longabaugh, R., Beattie, M., Noel, N., Stout, R., Malloy, P. (in press). The effect of social investment on treatment outcome. *Journal of Studies on Alcohol.*

Maisto, S.A., O'Farrell, T.J., Connors, G.J., McKay, J.R., & Pelcovits, M. (1988). Alcoholics' attributions of factors affecting their relapse to drinking and reasons for terminating relapse events following marital therapy. *Addictive Behaviors, 13*, 79-82.

Malcom, R., Anton, R.F., Randall, C.L., Johnston, A., Brady, K. & Theros, A. (1992). A placebo-controlled trial of Buspirone in anxious inpatient alcoholics. *Alcoholism: Clinical and Experimental Research, 16*, 1007-1013.

Marlatt, G.A., & Gordon, J.R. (1985). *Relapse prevention.* New York: Guilford Press.

McCrady, B.S. (1986). The family in the change process. In W. R. Miller & N. Heather (Eds.), *Treating addictive behaviors* (pp. 305-318). New York: Plenum.

McCrady, B.S., & Irvine, S. (1989). Self-help groups. In R.K. Hester & W.R. Miller (Eds.), *Handbook of alcoholism treatment approaches* (pp. 153-169). New York: Pergamon Press.

McCrady, B.S., Noel, N.E., Abrams, D.B., Stout, R.L., Nelson, H.F., & Hay, W.M. (1986). Comparative effectiveness of three types of spouse involvement in outpatient behavioral alcoholism treatment. *Journal of Studies on Alcohol, 47,* 459-467.

McCrady, B.S., & Irvine, S. (1989). Self-help groups. In R.K. Hester & W.R. Miller (Eds.), *Handbook of alcoholism treatment approaches,* (pp. 153-169). New York: Pergamon.

McKay, J.R., Alterman, A.I., McLellan, A.T., & Snider, E. (1993). *Inpatient versus day hospital rehabilitation for alcoholics: A comparison of experimental and nonexperimental designs.* Manuscript submitted for publication.

McKay, J.R., Alterman, A.I., McLellan, A.T., & Snider, E. (in press a). Day hospital substance abuse rehabilitation: Treatment goals, continuity of care, and outcome. *American Journal of Psychiatry.*

McKay, J.R., Longabaugh, R., Beattie, M.C., Maisto, S.A., & Noel, N. (1992). The relationship of pretreatment family functioning to drinking during follow-up by alcoholic patients. *American Journal of Drug and Alcohol Abuse, 18,* 445-460.

McKay, J.R., Longabaugh, R., Beattie, M.C., Maisto, S.A., & Noel, N. (in press b). Does adding conjoint therapy to individually-focused alcoholism treatment lead to better family functioning? *Journal of Substance Abuse.*

McKay, J.R., Longabaugh, R., Beattie, M.C., Maisto, S.A., & Noel, N. (in press d). Changes in family functioning during treatment and drinking outcomes for high and low autonomy alcoholics. *Addictive Behaviors.*

McKay, J.R., Maisto, S.A., & O'Farrell, T.J. (in press c). End-of-treatment self-efficacy, aftercare, and drinking outcomes of alcoholic men. *Alcoholism: Clinical and Experimental Research.*

McKay, J.R., McLellan, A.T., & Alterman, A.I. (1992). An evaluation of the Cleveland Criteria for inpatient substance abuse treatment. *American Journal of Psychiatry, 149,* 1212-1218.

McKay, J.R., Murphy, R., & Longabaugh, R. (1991). The effectiveness of alcoholism treatment: Evidence from outcome studies. In S.T. Mirin, J. Gossett, & M.C. Grob (Eds.), *Psychiatric treatment: Advances in outcome research* (pp. 143-158). Washington, D.C.: American Psychiatric Press, Inc.

McLachlan, J.F. (1972). Benefit from group therapy as a function of patient-therapist match on conceptual level. *Psychotherapy: Theory, Research, and Practice, 9,* 317-323.

McLachlan, J.F. (1974). Therapy strategies, personality orientation and recovery from alcoholism. *Canadian Psychiatric Association Journal, 19*, 25-30.

McLellan, A.T. (1986). "Psychiatric severity" as a predictor of outcome from substance abuse treatments. In R.E. Meyer (Ed.), *Psychopathology and addictive disorders* (pp. 97-139). New York: The Guilford Press.

McLellan, A.T., Luborsky L., Woody, G.E., & O'Brien C.P. (1980). An improved evaluation instrument for substance abuse patients: The Addiction Severity Index. *Journal of Nervous and Mental Disease, 168*, 26-33.

McLellan, A.T., Luborsky, L., Woody, G.E., Druley, K.A., & O'Brien, C.P. (1983). Predicting response to alcohol and drug abuse treatments: Role of psychiatric severity. *Archives of General Psychiatry, 40*, 620-625.

McLellan, A.T., Luborsky, L., O'Brien, C.P., Barr, H.L., & Evans, F. (1986). Alcohol and drug abuse treatment in three different populations: Is there improvement and is it predictable? *American Journal of Drug and Alcohol Abuse, 12*, 101-120.

McLellan, A.T., Woody, G.E., Luborsky, L., O'Brien, C.P., & Druley, K.A. (1983). Increased effectiveness of substance abuse treatment: A prospective study of patient-treatment "matching." *Journal of Nervous and Mental Disease, 171*, 597-605.

Miller, W.R. (1985). Motivation for treatment: A review with special emphasis on alcoholism. *Psychological Bulletin, 98*, 84-107.

Miller, W.R. (1992). Client/treatment matching in addictive behaviors. *The Behavior Therapist, 15*, 7-8.

Miller, W.R. (1989). Matching individual with interventions. In R.K. Hester & W.R. Miller (Eds.), *Handbook of alcoholism treatment approaches* (pp. 261-271). New York: Pergamon Press.

Miller, W.R., & Hester, R.K. (1986a). The effectiveness of alcoholism treatment: What research reveals. In W.R. Miller & N. Heather (Eds.), *Treating addictive behaviors: Process of change* (pp. 121-174), New York: Plenum.

Miller, W.R., & Hester, R.K. (1986b). Inpatient alcoholism treatment: Who benefits? *American Psychologist, 41*, 794-805.

Minkoff, K. (1991). Program components of a comprehensive integrated care system for serious mentally ill patients with substance disorders. In K. Minkoff & R. E. Drake (Eds.), *Dual diagnosis of major mental illness and substance disorder.* (pp. 12-28) San Francisco: Jossey-Bass, Inc.

Monti, P.M., Abrams, D.B., Binkoff, J.A., Zwick, W.R., Liepman, M.R., Nirenberg, T.D., & Rohsenow, D.J. (1990). Communication skills training, communication skills training with family, and cognitive behavioral mood management training for alcoholics. *Journal of Studies on Alcohol, 51*, 263-270.

Moos, R.H., Finney, J.W., & Cronkite, R.C. (1990). *Alcoholism treatment: Context, process, and outcome.* New York: Oxford University Press.

Moos, R.H., & Moos, B.S. (1984). The process of recovery from alcoholism: III. Comparing functioning in families of alcoholics and matched control families. *Journal of Studies on Alcohol, 45*, 111-118.

Nace, E.P. (1990). Inpatient treatment of alcoholism: A necessary part of the therapeutic armamentarium. *The Psychiatric Hospital, 21,* 9-31.

Noel, N.E., McCrady, B.S., Stout, R.L., & Fisher-Nelson, H. (1987). Predictors of attrition from an outpatient alcoholism treatment program for couples. *Journal of Studies on Alcohol, 48,* 229-235.

O'Farrell, T.J., Choquette, K.A., Cutter, H.S.G., Brown, E.D., & McCourt, W.F. (in press). Behavioral marital therapy with and without additional relapse prevention sessions for alcoholics and their wives. *Journal of Studies on Alcohol.*

O'Farrell, T.J., Cutter, H.S., Floyd, F.J. (1985). Evaluating behavioral marital therapy for male alcoholics: Effects on marital adjustment and communication from before to after treatment. *Behavior Therapy, 16,* 147-167.

Ojehagen, A., Berglund, M., Appel, G.P., Nilsson, B., & Skjaerris, A. (1990). Psychiatric symptoms in alcoholics attending outpatient treatment. *Alcoholism: Clinical and Experimental Research, 15,* 640-646.

Orford, J., Oppenheimer, E., & Edwards, G. (1976). Abstinence or control: The outcome for excessive drinkers two years after consultation. *Behavior Research and Therapy, 14,* 409-418.

Osher, F.C., & Kofoed, L.L. (1989). Treatment of patients with psychiatric and psychoactive substance abuse disorders. *Hospital and Community Psychiatry, 40,* 1025-1030.

Powell, B.J., Penick, E.C., Nickel, E.J., Liskow, B.I., Riesenmy, K.D., Campion, S.L., & Brown, E.F. (1992). Outcomes of co-morbid alcoholic men: A one-year follow-up. *Alcoholism: Clinical and Experimental Research, 16,* 131-138.

Prochaska, J.O., & DiClemente, C.C. (1992). Stages of change in the modification of problem behaviors. In M. Hersen, R.M. Eisler, & P.M. Miller (Eds.), *Progress in behavior modification* (Volume 28) (pp. 183-218). Sycamore, IL: Sycamore.

Prochaska, J.O., & DiClemente, C.C. (1986). Toward a comprehensive model of change. In W.R. Miller & N. Heather (Eds.), *Treating addictive behaviors: Process of change* (pp. 3-27). New York: Plenum.

Prochaska, J.O., DiClemente, C.C., & Norcross, J.C. (1992). In search of how people change: Applications to addictive behavior. *American Psychologist, 47,* 1102-1114.

Ridgely, M.S. (1991). Creating integrated programs for mentally ill persons with substance disorders. In K. Minkoff & R.E. Drake (Eds.), *Dual diagnosis of major mental illness and substance disorders* (pp. 29-41). San Francisco: Jossey-Bass, Inc.

Robins, L.N., Helzer, J.E., Przybeck, T.R., & Reiger, D.A. (1988). Alcohol disorders in the community: A report from the epidemiologic catchment area. In R.M. Rose & J. Barrett (Eds.), *Alcoholism: Origins and outcome* (pp. 15-29). New York: Raven Press.

Robins, L.N., Helzer, J.E., Weissman, M., Ovaschel, H., Gruenberg, E., Burke, J., & Regier, D.A. (1984). Lifetime prevalence of specific psychiatric disorders in three sites. *Archives of General Psychiatry, 38,* 381-389.

Rohsenow, D.J., Monti, P.M., Binkoff, J.A., Liepman, M.R., Nirenberg, T.D., & Abrams, D.B. (1991). Patient-treatment matching for alcoholic men in communication skills vs. cognitive-behavioral mood management training. *Addictive Behaviors, 16,* 63-69.

Rounsaville, B.J., Dolinsky, Z.S., Babor, T.F., & Meyer, R.E. (1987). Psychopathology as a predictor of treatment outcome in alcoholics. *Archives of General Psychiatry, 44,* 505-513.

Rounsaville, B.J., & Kleber, H.D. (1986). Psychiatric disorders in opiate addicts: Preliminary findings on the course and interaction with program type. In R.E. Meyer (Ed.), *Psychopathology and addictive disorders* (pp. 140-168). New York: The Guilford Press.

Saxe, L., Dougherty, D., Esty, K., & Fine, M. (1983). The effectiveness and costs of alcoholism treatment. *Health Technology Case Study #22,* Washington: Government Printing Office.

Schuckit, M.A. (1985). The clinical implications of primary diagnostic groups among alcoholics. *Archives of General Psychiatry, 42,* 1043-1049.

Smith, D.I. (1985). Evaluation of a residential AA program for women. *Alcohol and Alcoholism, 20,* 315-327.

Smith, D.I. (1986). Evaluation of a residential AA program. *International Journal of the Addictions, 21,* 33-49.

Sobell, L.C., Maisto, S.A., Sobell, M.B., & Cooper, A.M. (1979). Reliability of alcohol abusers' self-reports of drinking behavior. *Behavior Research and Therapy, 17,* 157-160.

Stout, R.L., McCrady, B.S., Longabaugh, R., Noel, N.E., & Beattie, M.C. (1989). *Marital therapy helps maintain then effectiveness of alcohol treatment: Replication of an outcome crossover effect.* Unpublished manuscript.

Vaillant, G.E. (1983). *The natural history of alcoholism.* Cambridge MA: Harvard University Press.

Volpicelli, J.R., Alterman, A.I., Hayashida, M., & O'Brien, C.P. (1992). Naltrexone in the treatment of alcohol dependence. *Archives of General Psychiatry, 49,* 876-880.

Walsh, D.C., Hingson, R.W., Merrigan, D.M., Morelock Levenson, S., Cupples, A., Heeren, T., Coffman, G.A., Becker, C.A., Barker, T.A., Hamilton, S.K., McGuire, T.G., & Kelly, C.A. (1991). A randomized trial of treatment options for alcohol-abusing workers. *New England Journal of Medicine, 325,* 775-782.

Weiss, R., and Mirin, S. (1987). Substance abuse as an attempt at self-medication. *Psychiatric Medicine, 3,* 357-367.

# Recent Developments in Detection and Biological Indicators of Alcoholism

## Arthur W. K. Chan, PhD

**SUMMARY.** Although doctors are uniquely placed to detect hazardous or harmful drinking and alcoholism, much research has documented that these problems are underdiagnosed in clinical settings. This paper summarizes recent developments of easy-to-use and brief questionnaires that health professionals can use to screen patients for heavy drinking/alcoholism. These instruments can be combined with laboratory indicators of the metabolic and biochemical effects of excessive alcohol consumption. New biochemical indicators of alcoholism as well as recent investigations of biological indicators of vulnerability (trait markers) to develop alcoholism are also reviewed. This information, together with the reasons why health professionals need to be involved in screening patients for alcohol abuse/alcoholism, should be included in medical education curriculum and continuing education programs.

## INTRODUCTION

It has been well documented that alcohol abuse and alcoholism are associated with increased morbidity and mortality (German,

---

Arthur W. K. Chan is affiliated with the Research Institute on Addictions, New York State Office of Alcoholism and Substance Abuse Services, 1021 Main Street, Buffalo, NY 14203.

Arthur W. K. Chan thanks Janet Berg for her skillful preparation of the manuscript.

[Haworth co-indexing entry note]: "Recent Developments in Detection and Biological Indicators of Alcoholism," Chan, Arthur W.K. Co-published simultaneously in *Drugs & Society* (The Haworth Press, Inc.) Vol. 8, No. 1, 1993, pp. 31-67; and: *Innovations in Alcoholism Treatment: State of the Art Reviews and Their Implications for Clinical Practice* (ed: Gerard J. Connors) The Haworth Press, Inc., 1993, pp. 31-67. Multiple copies of this article/chapter may be purchased from The Haworth Document Delivery Center [1-800-3-HAWORTH; 9:00 a.m. - 5:00 p.m. (EST)].

1973; Klatsky et al., 1981; Kolb & Gunderson, 1983; Smith & Kraus, 1988; Umbricht-Schneiter & Santora, 1991). Therefore, alcohol researchers have emphasized the importance of early identification of excessive drinking and alcoholism in minimizing the adverse medical, social, and economic consequences of various alcohol-related problems. Although doctors are uniquely placed to detect alcohol-related problems and to provide interventions, much research has documented that doctors fail to identify the majority of their patients with drinking problems (Bradley, 1992; Chan, 1990; Moore et al., 1989; Schuckit & Irwin, 1988). Anderson (1992) has provided a thorough summary of the reasons why doctors need to be involved in screening their patients for heavy drinking/alcohol abuse. Reports of prevalence of alcoholism in patients of hospital clinics have ranged 4 to 70% (e.g., Baird, 1989; Conigrave, 1991; Hiller et al., 1989), with the majority being 20 to 25%. The wide variations in prevalence were due to different gold standards used for the definition of alcoholism/alcohol abuse, different diagnostic instruments used, and the types of clinics studied. Even among different departments within a hospital, there were reported differences in doctors' abilities and willingness to identify alcoholism and alcohol abuse in their patients, e.g., 7% for gynecology, 27% for surgery, and 67% for psychiatry (Moore et al., 1989). Several factors can contribute to the underdiagnosis of alcoholism by doctors: inadequate training, especially in obtaining historical information about alcohol-related problems and on how to integrate historical information, medical symptoms, and laboratory data to arrive at diagnosis; lack of understanding of the usual course of alcoholism; erroneous stereotyping of alcoholics; alcoholism being viewed by some doctors as not within the realm of medical treatment; and patients underreporting their alcohol consumption (Dobkin et al., 1991; Schuckit, 1987). Many clinicians do not think that patients' self-reports of alcohol consumption can be used as reliable tools in the detection of early alcohol abuse (Eckardt et al., 1986). Therefore, they may prefer more objective methods such as biochemical tests or physical symptoms.

Research on the detection of alcoholism over the last two decades has primarily involved the use of specific questionnaires aimed at eliciting information about alcohol-related problems and patterns/amounts of alcohol consumption in respondents, or laboratory tests as indicators of physiological damage resulting from chronic heavy alcohol intake. In many instances, a combination of both approaches was used. This paper provides an update of investigations using these two detection strategies, with particular emphasis on the use of brief questionnaires and the more recently proposed biological indicators of alcoholism.

## SCREENING QUESTIONNAIRES

Because doctors generally have busy schedules, they may be reluctant to spend time administering lengthy questionnaires or to personally conduct a structured interview. Even the completion of a self-administered questionnaire by patients in the waiting room may be considered by some doctors as potentially upsetting to their patients, especially if the questionnaire contains mainly alcohol-related questions. Contrary to this belief, the experience of investigators in the World Health Organization (WHO) Collaborative Project on the identification and treatment of persons with harmful alcohol consumption indicated that many patients who were heavy drinkers were pleased to find that a health worker was interested in their use of alcohol and the problems associated with it (Babor et al., 1989). For patients who may be uncooperative or defensive, a health survey questionnaire in which some alcohol-specific questions are embedded is preferred. Doctors may also feel that they will be put in an awkward position of having to provide counseling about their patients' alcohol abuse problems and to provide referral for treatment. These actions are not generally considered by doctors to be part of routine medical treatment. Such attitudes are unfortunate because several studies have shown that brief and early interventions by general practitioners can have a significant impact on the overall prevention of excessive alcohol intake and alcoholism (Anderson, 1992; Saunders & Foulds, 1992; Scott & Anderson, 1990; Wallace et al., 1988). Therefore, it is imperative that alcoholism screening questionnaires be brief and easily administered by health professionals.

The importance of appropriate phrasing in alcohol-use questions is illustrated by the study of Cyr and Wartman (1988) in which the questions "How much do you drink?" and "How often do you drink?" yielded low sensitivities of 34.0% and 46.8%, respectively, in identifying alcoholic patients in an ambulatory medical clinic. The patients were designated as alcoholics based on their scores on the Michigan Alcoholism Screening Test (MAST). On the other hand, the question "Have you ever had a drinking problem?" had a sensitivity of 70.2% and when it was combined with "When was your last drink?" (using drinking within the preceding 24 hours as the alcoholic response), it had a sensitivity of 91.5% and a specificity of 89.7% (Cyr & Wartman, 1988). Using this instrument to screen for alcoholism in an academic, general medicine clinic, Goldberg et al. (1991) reported that 35.6% of the patients screened were found to be positive. More importantly, over four times as many patients screened this way (10.8% vs. 2.3%) accepted referrals for counseling, as did patients seen by doctors providing standard care. Studies of elderly veterans and women have indicated that this test was less useful in these populations (Bradley, 1992; Moran et al., 1990). This two-item instrument appears to be useful as a primary screening tool for alcoholism in clinical settings, although more research is needed to evaluate thoroughly its effectiveness in different clinical populations.

The CAGE, a four-item questionnaire, is an acronym for: *Cut* down on drinking, *Annoyed* by criticism of drinking, feeling *Guilty* about drinking, *Eye-opener* (morning drinking). Two or more positive responses are indicative of problem drinking or probable alcoholism (Ewing, 1984). The advantages of the CAGE are its brevity and high clinical validity (Smart et al., 1991). Thus, many studies have shown that the CAGE identified most alcoholics and excessive drinkers (Buchsbaum et al., 1991; Bush et al., 1987; Ewing, 1984; Mayfield et al., 1974; Pileire et al., 1991). However, some studies have reported relatively low sensitivity for the CAGE in other selected populations, such as college students, DWI offenders, emergency room patients, and elderly medical patients (Barrett & Vaughan Williams, 1989; Bernadt et al., 1984; Heck & Lichtenberg, 1990; Mangion et al., 1992; Mischke & Venneri, 1987). The disadvantages of the CAGE are that it focuses on lifetime rather than current problems. Therefore, it cannot distinguish past problem drinkers or alcoholics who are currently abstinent from those who have relapsed and are current heavy drinkers. Moreover, the questions about "cutting down" and "feeling guilty" are often answered positively by current light drinkers, especially those who had misspent youth (Kent, 1991). For this reason, there may be an overestimation of alcohol-related problems by the CAGE (Rydon et al., 1992). The data in Table 1 illustrate the importance of including a recency (e.g., past year) criterion for positive CAGE responses. In this study (Chan, unpublished data), the CAGE was part of a questionnaire administered to male and female alcoholics in a county hospital treatment center and to clinical outpatients in the same hospital. Although 42.6% of the clinical outpatients tested lifetime positive, only 16.9% of them met the one-year recency criterion. On the other hand, there was no significant difference in the percentage of alcoholics tested positive on the CAGE for lifetime and for past year problems, a result consistent with the fact that the alcoholics were being treated for current problems. Those clinical outpatients not meeting the one-year recency criterion could be recovering alcoholics who were either abstinent or relatively light drinkers not currently having alcohol-related problems, current light drinkers who were false positives because of the inherent phrasing problems of the CAGE alluded to above, or current light drinkers who were previously heavy drinkers or had few alcohol related problems in the past, but were never alcoholics. It is to be expected that light drinkers (males < 3 drinks/day and females < 2 drinks/day) would have the largest percentage of false positives and that they would have the borderline CAGE score of two. Our results (unpublished) indeed indicate that among those fitting the foregoing criteria, near-

TABLE 1. Percentage of Subjects Tested Positive Using the CAGE

| History | Alcoholics (N = 185) | Clinical Outpatients (N = 281) |
|---------|----------------------|--------------------------------|
| Lifetime | 97.2 | 42.6 |
| ≤ 1 year* | 94.4 | 16.9 |

* Current age minus age when the alcohol-related problems occurred the last time

ly 70% were false positives and they were only lifetime CAGE positives but not for past year. There has been only one study that used the CAGE in a general population survey of drinking (Smart et al., 1991). Therefore, more research is needed to validate the utility of the CAGE in general population surveys.

A variant of the CAGE is the T-ACE questionnaire (Sokol et al., 1989) in which three of the items in the CAGE were retained, namely, A, C, E. T stands for tolerance to alcohol, which was defined as > 2 drinks to make a female subject feel "high." The rationale for asking about tolerance to the inebriating effect of alcohol is that it does not trigger denial and may be useful for detecting alcohol abuse (Sokol et al., 1989). For this reason, a weighted score of two was given for a positive response to T, and one point for the three other questions (A, C, E), with a total score of $\geq 2$ being considered positive. The T-ACE was used in the prenatal detection of risk-drinking in gravid women, and it correctly identified 69% of the at-risk drinkers (Sokol et al., 1989). Its validity needs to be further investigated in other clinical populations. Other variations of the T-ACE and CAGE are the 3-item NET (N, normal drinker; E, eye-opener; T, tolerance) and the 5-item TWEAK (T, tolerance; W, worry about drinking; E, eye-opener; A, amnesia from drinking; K/C, cut down) (Russell et al., 1991). Tolerance in both instruments was defined either as the number of drinks needed to get high ( $\geq 3$ drinks) or the number of drinks one could hold ( $\geq 5$ drinks). Therefore, theoretically there are two versions of each instrument. Because discriminant analysis indicated that "Tolerance" and "Worry" contributed more to the prediction of risk-drinking in women than the other items, these two items were given a weighted score of two, while the other items each had a 1-point score (Russell et al., 1991). Scores of 2+ were positive on the NET and scores of 3+ positive on the TWEAK. When applied to the screening of risk-drinking in pregnant women, the TWEAK and T-ACE versions and the NET (hold) had sensitivity ranging from 68-89% and specificity from 80-93%. However, the NET (high) had a 100% sensitivity but only 22% specificity (Russell et al., 1991). Our preliminary investigations using the TWEAK as part of a questionnaire found that its sensitivity/specificity was 94.4%/- for alcoholics in treatment; 92.3%/89.3% for clinical outpatients; and 89.1%/68.5% for a general population sample.

The 25-item Michigan Alcoholism Screening Test (MAST) (Selzer, 1971) is the parent of another family of closely related tests such as the 10-item brief MAST (Pokorny et al., 1972), the 13-item short MAST (Selzer et al., 1975), the self-administered alcoholism screening test (SAAST) (Swenson & Morse, 1975), and the Malmo MAST (Mm-MAST) (Kristenson & Trell, 1982). Many of the questions in these similar tests deal with late stages of severe alcohol abuse; for example, whether the patient has attended Alcoholics Anonymous or has been admitted to a hospital because of drinking. Therefore, they may not be sufficiently sensitive in detecting early stages of alcohol abuse. Another drawback is that many of the questions focus on lifetime problems. Thus, in our study (unpublished) using the brief MAST to detect alcohol abuse/alcoholism in clinical outpatients, the results parallel those involving the use of CAGE (Table 1) in that 33.8% of the outpatients tested lifetime positive in brief MAST, but the percentage decreased to 19.5% upon inclusion of the past-year criterion. Moreover, nearly 90% of those who were lifetime positive (but not past-year) on the brief MAST with borderline scores of 6 to 9 but who reported to be light drinkers (see previous definition) in the past year, were false positives.

The Alcohol Use Disorders Identification Test (AUDIT) was designed for the early detection of harmful drinking in primary health care settings, but it can also detect alcoholism with a high degree of accuracy (Babor et al., 1989). The main screening instrument is a ten-item questionnaire containing alcohol-specific questions, three on the amount and frequency of drinking, three on alcohol dependence, and four on adverse consequences of alcohol. Nine of the ten questions are scored 0-4 each and one question is scored 0-5, depending on the responses, with a highest possible score of 41. The WHO recommends a total score of 11 or more as suggestive of a drinking problem. The distinctive features of the AUDIT are: (a) it is specifically designed for international uses; (b) it is brief, rapid and flexible; (c) it focuses on recent alcohol use; (d) it is consistent with the International Classification of Diseases Criteria (ICD-10); (e) it identifies harmful and hazardous alcohol use rather than alcoholism; (f) it also contains a supplementary nonalcohol-specific clinical screening instrument that consists of two questions about traumatic injury, five items on clinical examination, and a blood test on serum gamma-glutamyltransferase (GGT) activity (Babor et al., 1989). This latter instrument is recommended in situations in which alcohol-specific questions may not be reliably answered. Fleming et al. (1991) applied the AUDIT in a sample of college students using DSM-III criteria for alcohol abuse as the gold standard. They reported that AUDIT had a sensitivity of 84% and a specificity of 71% when the recommended cutoff score of 11 was used. The study indicated that a large percentage (29%) of the college students met DSM-III criteria for alcohol abuse, with blackouts and drinking six or more drinks on one occasion being the most discriminating features between problem and nonproblem drinking groups. Further testing of AUDIT for its validity and reliability in other populations with a wider age range needs to be conducted. It also will be important to use other diagnostic interview criteria to confirm the findings of Fleming et al. (1991).

The "Alcohol Clinical Index" or ACI (Skinner & Holt, 1987; Skinner et al., 1986) is another potentially useful instrument designed for use by doctors to screen patients for alcohol abuse or alcoholism. The unique features of this instrument are that it combines clinical signs, medical history, laboratory tests and alcohol questionnaires. These are categorized into two components, a 17-item Clinical Signs checklist and a 13-item Medical History questionnaire. Initial testing of the ACI in alcoholics, social drinkers, and nonalcoholic family practice outpatients (Skinner et al., 1986) indicated that the ACI identified alcoholics better than did laboratory indicators. The investigators suggested that there was a need to further evaluate the ACI in other populations. However, no widespread validation of the ACI study has appeared in the literature. An exception was a study by Alterman et al. (1992), who used the ACI in lower socioeconomic alcoholics in an outpatient medical clinic at a VA Medical Center. They found that the Clinical Signs checklist had high sensitivity but poor specificity, with an overall accuracy of 70%. The Medical History questionnaire had 100% specificity but more moderate sensitivity using a cutoff score of two or more. The limitations of the study were its small sample and extreme differences between the alcoholics and nonalcoholics (Alterman et al., 1992). Therefore, it remains to be determined whether the ACI can easily differentiate less severe alcoholics from a broad range of social drinkers.

## BIOCHEMICAL INDICATORS

Traditionally genetic markers of diseases denote enduring heritable traits with known patterns of inheritance. However, the term "marker," as commonly used in alcohol research, has the same meaning as "indicator," and a true genetic marker of alcoholism has yet to be found (Hill et al., 1987). Nevertheless, for convenience of referring to published data, "marker" is used synonymously with "indicator" in this paper. The categorization of alcoholism markers into trait (vulnerability) and state markers separates biochemical indices of vulnerability to develop alcoholism from biochemical changes resulting from chronic and excessive alcohol intake, respectively. The pros and cons of conventional state markers as well as recent studies on trait markers have been reviewed in detail elsewhere (Chan, 1990; Crabb, 1990; Cushman et al., 1984; Eckardt et al., 1986; Eskay & Linnoila, 1991; Holt et al., 1981; Lumeng, 1986; Mihas & Tavassoli, 1992; Rosman & Lieber, 1990; Salaspuro, 1986; Schuckit, 1986; Watson et al., 1986). Therefore, the focus of this paper is on recent developments in trait and state markers of alcoholism.

*Trait (Vulnerability) Markers.* Investigations through 1990 have been reviewed elsewhere (Begleiter & Porjesz, 1988; Chan, 1990, 1991; Crabb, 1990; Eskay & Linnoila, 1991; Schuckit, 1992; Tabakoff & Hoffman, 1988). Methodological considerations in studies of populations at high risk for alcoholism have also been reviewed (Chan, 1990; Schuckit, 1992). A major portion of earlier studies has been focused on baseline differences between subjects with a positive history of familial alcoholism (FHP) and those with a negative history of familial alcoholism (FHN). Such differences include a reduced $P_3$ (or P300) amplitude of the event-related potential (ERP), differential beta or alpha activity in the EEG, possible differences in Monoamine Oxidase activity, and possible cognitive, behavioral and neurological deficits in FHP subjects (Chan, 1990;

Schuckit, 1992; Tarter et al., 1990). Recently, Whipple et al. (1991) reported that, compared to FHN subjects, FHP subjects exhibited increased latency and decreased amplitude $P_3$ in the ERP for a difficult task (but not for an easy task). These results might explain some of the earlier inconsistent findings. Other studies involved comparisons between FHP and FHN subjects in their acute responses to alcohol. Based on initial findings (Moss et al., 1989; O'Malley & Maisto, 1985; Pollock et al., 1986; Schuckit, 1980, 1984) showing that FHP subjects were less sensitive to the acute effects of ethanol than FHN subjects, it was speculated that such differences might be the basis for the increased risk in developing alcohol-related problems in FHP individuals because they need to consume more alcohol to achieve their desired drug effect. The finding that there was a greater stress-dampening effect from ethanol in FHP subjects also supported this speculation (Levenson et al., 1987). However, there have been reports that FHP subjects exhibited greater psychomotor impairment by ethanol and that there were no differences in subjective ratings of ethanol effects among FHP and FHN subjects (Vogel-Sprott & Chipperfield, 1987; Wilson & Nagoshi, 1988). But these studies involved administration of alcohol over a period of 1 hour or longer and they may not be directly comparable to earlier studies which involved oral or intravenous infusion of alcohol over 10 minutes (Schuckit, 1992). The same inconsistencies have persisted in more recent reports. McCaul et al. (1990) reported that FHP subjects had significantly greater responses on a variety of subjective effects of ethanol than FHN subjects. De Wit and McCracken (1990) found that there were no differences between FHP and FHN subjects either in the frequency of choice of ethanol over placebo or in the total dose of ethanol self-administration. The two groups also did not differ on most measures of acute ethanol effects, such as mood-altering effects or behavioral changes. However, this study was criticized for the low blood alcohol levels and a small intensity of alcohol effect (Schuckit, 1992). Newlin and Thomson (1991) suggested that the discrepancies in the comparisons of acute effects of ethanol in FHP and FHN subjects might be due to the inability of a simple alcohol challenge to distinguish between sensitivity to alcohol, acute tolerance, chronic tolerance, and interactions of the alcohol response with the novelty of the laboratory environment. A study of a national sample of college students (Engs, 1990) showed that having a positive family background for heavy drinking was not associated with either light or heavy alcohol consumption. But it should be emphasized that these students were categorized as having a positive or negative family background of possible problem drinking, but not a positive or negative family history of alcoholism as classified by the DSM-III criteria. On the other hand, some recent findings have provided rational explanation for the increased risk of developing alcoholism in first degree relatives of alcoholics, and for the earlier onset and more severe course of alcoholism in these individuals, as suggested by earlier studies (Worobec et al., 1990). Thus, Newlin and Pretorius (1990) found that sons of alcoholics reported significantly greater hangover symptoms in the past year than sons of nonalcoholics, with the two groups reporting comparable quantity/frequency of recent drinking. Alcoholics who were FHP were more reliant on alcohol to manage moods and were relatively insensitive to negative consequences compared to alcoholics who were FHN (Worobec et al., 1990); these differences might theoretically account for the vulnerability to more severe alcoholism in the FHP alcoholics.

Earlier reports indicate that there were differential responses to a challenge dose of ethanol among FHP and FHN subjects such as changes in hormonal levels such as prolactin, cortisol, and adrenocorticotropic hormone. Recently Lex et al. (1991) reported that FHP women had significantly lower prolactin levels 40 to 80 minutes following 0.56g/kg alcohol compared to FHN women. The results replicated findings reported by Schuckit et al. (1987b) that FHP men had lower prolactin levels than FHN men following the ingestion of a higher dose of alcohol (0.83g/kg). In contrast, FHP women had higher cortisol levels than FHN women 110 to 130 minutes after alcohol (Lex et al, 1991) whereas FHP men had lower cortisol levels than FHN men following alcohol (Schuckit et al., 1987a). Conflicting results have also been reported for the thyrotropin response to intravenous thyrotropin-releasing hormone (TRH) in FHP and FHN subjects, with reports of no difference between the two groups (Monteiro et al., 1990), or increased incidences of a blunted TSH response to TRH in FHP subjects (Loosen et al., 1987). More recent biochemical studies include demonstrations that FHP subjects had a significantly higher mean Vmax but not Km for platelet serotonin uptake (Rausch et al., 1991), and less plasma GABA-like activity which was normalized by alcohol intake (Moss et al., 1990), than in FHN subjects. Hill et al. (1991) found no significant differences in baseline membrane fluidity or on the fluidizing effects of ethanol between FHP and FHN subjects.

As yet there have been no formal reports of follow-up studies of FHP and FHN subjects tested in the investigations summarized above. Such follow-up studies could help determine the relationship between the potential vulnerability markers and development of alcoholism; they also could provide information about how these markers and/or family history of alcoholism might relate to future problems with alcohol as well as other drugs, and to major mental disorders (Schuckit, 1992). Preliminary results of follow-ups of 100 such individuals suggest that "the rate of severe alcohol-related life difficulties appears to be approximately three times as high in the FHPs, and there is a trend showing increased levels of severe life problems related to cocaine and marijuana in these men at high risk for alcoholism" (Schuckit, 1992). Additionally, those FHPs who were alcohol dependent at some period during the follow-up had significantly lower levels of intensity of response to alcohol at the time of initial testing compared to FHPs who did not develop alcohol dependence (Schuckit, 1992). More detailed analysis of data from the follow-up of more than 400 subjects is expected to be available in 1996 (Schuckit, 1992).

The similar pharmacological actions between ethanol and the benzodiazepines prompted investigations to test whether the differential responses to ethanol seen in FHP and FHN subjects could be generalized to other depressant drugs such as diazepam. Schuckit et al. (1991b) found that unlike the reactions to ethanol, levels of cortisol, prolactin, and growth hormone were not significantly different in FHP and FHN subjects following an intravenous infusion of diazepam. Likewise, the two groups did not differ in subjective feelings and changes in body sway following diazepam (Schuckit et al., 1991a). Using a double-blind preference procedure in which subjects first sampled diazepam and placebo and then chose the substance they preferred, De Wit (1991) found that neither the FHP nor the FHN group chose diazepam more often than placebo. Both groups also did not differ in their responses to diazepam, such as subjective drug effects or drug liking. These data are in contrast to those of Ciraulo et al. (1989), who found that FHP subjects exhibited a greater euphorgenic response to alprazolam than FHN subjects. However, the Ciraulo study was criticized for the lack of a placebo control and because the FHP group had higher average alcohol use in the 6 months prior to the study than did the FHN group. Ethanol and secobarbital produced comparable impairment in FHP and FHN subjects for most psychomotor responses (McCaul et al., 1990), but in this study, FHP subjects reported greater subjective effects of ethanol than FHN subjects at equivalent blood alcohol levels. Following a high dose of secobarbital (200 mg), FHP but not FHN subjects showed elevated subjective effects, but the magnitudes were substantially less than those observed following ethanol (McCaul et al., 1990). In another study, McCaul et al. (1991) found that FHP subjects reported more extended intoxication and greater withdrawal effects following both ethanol and the high dose of secobarbital than did FHN subjects. Taken together, the data suggest that FHP subjects may react to ethanol differently compared to FHN subjects, and that such differences may only partially generalize to other drug classes. It will be of interest to extend the studies of McCaul et al. (1990, 1991) to other drugs such as marijuana and cocaine.

Another very important area of research over the past several years has been centered on the identification of specific genes that influence the risk or expression of alcoholism. There has been suggestive evidence in earlier reports that there were possible linkages between alcoholism and genes on chromosomes 4 and 13, but replications of these studies have not been performed (Hill et al., 1988; Tanna et al., 1988). Tabakoff et al. (1988) showed that platelet adenylate cyclase (AC) activity, when stimulated by agents such as cesium fluoride, was significantly lowered among alcoholics compared with nonalcoholics. They suggested that it might be a trait marker of alcoholism. This work and that of Diamond et al. (1987), who found low receptor-activated AC activity in the lymphocytes of alcoholics, prompted Devor et al. (1991) to investigate the genetics of AC activity. Although the investigators detected a major Mendelian effect in fluoride-stimulated platelet AC activity, they found no correlation between such AC activity and alcoholism status. This result casts doubt that there is relationship between the stimulated AC activity and vulnerability to alcoholism, but it is possible that the samples were too heterogeneous for cosegregation to be detected (Devor et al., 1991).

The role of the $D_2$ dopamine receptor gene in alcoholism has been examined, beginning with the study by Blum et al. (1990) that suggested that the $A_1$ allele of the $D_2$ dopamine receptor gene was associated with a severe form of alcoholism. These initial findings were viewed with skepticism (Gordis et al., 1990) because of the following: (a) sketchy clinical description of the alcoholic and non-alcoholic subjects; (b) alcoholism was diagnosed retrospectively after deaths from a variety of causes; (c) unclear definition of a "virulent type" of alcoholism with which the $A_1$ allele was associated. Since then there have been reports supporting (Blum et al., 1991; Bolos et al., 1990; Noble et al., 1991; Parsian et al., 1991; Uhl et al., 1992) and refuting the seminal findings of Blum et al. (Comings et al., 1991; Cook et al., 1992; Gelernter et al., 1991; Turner et al., 1992). The studies up to 1991 have been reviewed by Cloninger (1991), who concluded that "the findings of an allelic association with alcoholism in the absence of tight linkage supports the hypothesis that the $A_1$ allele modifies clinical expression, but is neither a necessary or sufficient cause of alcoholism." Another review of these data (Uhl et al., 1992) also supports the association between the dopamine $D_2$ receptor alleles and substance abuse, not just alcoholism. The findings that alcoholics had reduced dopamine receptor sensitivity and binding characteristics (Balldin et al., 1992; Noble et al., 1991) cannot distinguish whether such abnormalities are genetically determined or acquired after long-term alcohol consumption. Two recent reports (Cook et al., 1992; Turner et al., 1992) both used alcoholics with severe alcoholism (based on duration of alcohol-related problems, heavy alcohol intake, and medical complications of alcoholism) and did not find any significant relationship between alcoholism severity and $A_1$ allele frequency, contrary to the work of Blum et al. (1990). One speculative explanation of the conflicting results is that the two recent studies tended to exclude subjects who had antisocial personality traits and/or primary psychiatric disorders. The work of Comings et al. (1991) and the review of Cloninger (1991) both suggested that the $A_1$ allele might serve a modifier role rather than the cause in the expression of alcoholism, and might be a marker for personality characteristics conducive to drug abuse behavior. Therefore, future investigations need to evaluate additional behavioral pathologies to which the $A_1$ allele might predispose (Uhl et al., 1991) and the influences of environmental factors. As Turner et al. (1992) have cautioned, "association studies are highly vulnerable to subtle biases in populations; therefore, in studies of this type, vigorous characterization of a large sample of subjects and controls is necessary, including examination of the subjects' ethnicity to avoid spurious associations generated by alleles that differ in frequency between ethnic groups." The list of potential candidate genes in alcoholism (Devor & Cloninger, 1989) will undoubtedly grow and be refined as more investigators incorporate the latest techniques of molecular biology in their searches for trait markers for alcoholism.

## Conventional State Markers

Although ethanol is the only true indicator of alcohol consumption, its usefulness is limited by its relatively rapid elimination. Other disadvantages include the inability to consistently detect binge drinkers and to distinguish acute from chronic alcohol intake. Despite these limitations, determinations of the level of ethanol in blood, urine, or breath can provide meaningful information under certain settings, such as emergency hospital admissions, monitoring of alcoholism treatment programs, alcohol-related violence in victims as well as in perpetrators, and drunk-driving offenses. Because of the development of tolerance to alcohol in chronic heavy drinkers, it has been recommended that a blood alcohol level (BAL) exceeding 150 mg/dl in a patient without gross evidence of intoxication strongly suggests alcohol abuse (National Council on Alcoholism, 1972). Likewise, a BAL higher than 300 mg/dl recorded at any time, or a level higher than 100 mg/dl recorded during a routine medical examination, can be considered as a strong indicator of alcoholism (National Council on Alcoholism, 1972). A recent study (Wieczorek et al., 1992) on drinking and driving offenders found no significant relationship between BAL and alcohol abuse or dependence diagnoses or between problem drinking and BAL. Thus, the usefulness of a single report of BAL for diagnostic screening purposes may be limited. Olsen et al. (1989) reported that ethanol elimination rates (EER) determined by serial breath analyses had a higher sensitivity and specificity than other conventional markers for the detection of ethanol consumption above the limit of 50 g per day. They found that 13 out of 15 alcoholics had EER higher than the highest EER found in the control group, confirming earlier reports of elevated EER among chronic drinkers (Katerer et al., 1969; Ugarte et al., 1977). However, the usefulness of this test is contingent upon the recent consumption of ethanol in individuals being tested. Otherwise, the ethical dilemma of having to administer alcohol to alcoholics or problem drinkers needs to be contended with. Analysis of urinary levels of ethanol during abstinence appears to be an attractive alternative to the determination of BAL for recent excessive alcohol consumption. This method requires the use of sophisticated instruments, namely a combination of gas chromatograph and mass spectrometry (GC/MS). Using such a method, Tang (1987, 1991) reported that even after 14 days of abstinence, urinary ethanol was significantly higher in abstaining alcoholics than in social drinkers. The source of ethanol in urine was from ethanol conjugates formed during alcohol consumption (Tang, 1991). The usefulness of this test for screening purposes can be questioned because of the potential confounding effect of recent acute alcohol intake prior to urine samples being collected. A urinary alcohol-specific product, which has an unknown chemical identity (presumably a breakdown product of acetaldehyde-protein adduct), has been found to be increased 17 times in chronic alcoholics compared to controls (Tang et al., 1986). However, no recent investigation has appeared to confirm or refute the usefulness of this proposed marker of alcoholism.

Among the many conventional state markers of alcoholism, the two most often used in clinical studies are gamma-glutamyltransferase (GGT) and mean corpuscular volume (MCV). Seppa et al. (1992) suggested that MCV might not be the only hematologic parameter showing abnormality in alcoholics, and that high red cell distribution width was even more common among alcoholics than high MCV. The possibility of red cell distribution width as a new marker for alcoholism needs to be investigated. Other popular tests include serum levels of the liver enzymes aspartate aminotransferase (ASAT or SGOT) and alanine aminotransferase (ALAT or SGPT). These markers by themselves lack sufficient sensitivity to be reliable markers of alcoholism or to be used as screening tests for heavy alcohol consumption because elevated activities are also found in many diseases or drug therapies unrelated to alcohol intake (Chan, 1990; Chick et al., 1981; Latcham, 1986; Seppa et al., 1992). Nevertheless, doctors can use an abnormal test result as a reason for questioning a patient's drinking more closely. This is especially important in light of reports suggesting that brief and early interventions by doctors can have a significant impact on the prevention of alcohol abuse and alcoholism (Saunders & Foulds, 1992; Scott & Anderson, 1990; Wallace et al., 1988). Unfortunately, physicians were parsimonious in ordering these tests (Graham, 1991). Teoh et al. (1992) reported that over 60% of alcohol-dependent or polysubstance-dependent women of reproductive age and over 80% of alcohol-dependent women of postmenopausal age had either increased MCV or hyperprolactinemia. There are conflicting reports concerning the usefulness of MCV or GGT in detecting alcohol abuse during pregnancy (Barrison et al., 1982; Halmesmaki et al., 1992; Ylikorkala et al., 1987). Because of the prevalence of multiple drug use in alcoholics (Chan, 1991), there is a need to consider the influences of concomitant drug use in the study of state markers of alcoholism. As an example, Chang et al. (1990) found that alcoholics who also used other drugs had significantly lower MCV and GGT values than subjects who used alcohol alone; specifically, cocaine use was associated with lower MCV values, marijuana use with lower ASAT values, and heroin use with high ASAT and GGT values. These differences between drug-using and nondrug-using alcoholics were still significant even after controlling for age and quantity, frequency and duration of alcohol consumption (Chang et al., 1990). The above popular laboratory tests have also been used as adjunctive monitoring of treatment effectiveness and relapses of drinking since the elevated enzyme activities usually decreased upon abstinence and reelevated upon resumption of alcohol drinking (Keso & Salaspuro, 1990a, 1990b; Orrego et al., 1985). However, Orrego et al. (1985) suggested that because of the prolonged half-life of serum GGT decay in alcoholics who remained abstinent, individual variations in serum GGT levels during treatment should be interpreted with caution. This is because a drop in GGT does not preclude the possibility of relapse, and conversely, an elevated level does not preclude abstinence.

*Combination Tests.* Earlier investigations have demonstrated that combinations of a large number of tests have generally yielded better results than single tests or combinations of a few tests (Chan, 1990). The use of discriminant function analyses of laboratory test batteries was first reported by Ryback et al. (1980, 1982), who found excellent classifications between severe alcoholics and abstainers based on the profiles of 24 laboratory tests. Subsequent studies using similar methods but with less impaired or young alcoholics and other selected populations (Beresford et al., 1988; Chan, 1990) also reported fairly high sensitivity (74%-99%). However, less successful results have also been reported (Chan, 1990; Beresford et al., 1990). Vanclay et al. (1991) reported that a discriminant function analysis of a battery of blood chemistry tests together with body weight, smoking status and systolic blood pressure, had a sensitivity of 78% in classifying high alcohol consumption in a community sample of adult males. One major disadvantage of the discriminant function analysis (or other statistical methods such as regression analysis) of a large panel of laboratory tests is that the accuracy of classification is dependent on a precise separation of the groups under study. Thus, inaccurate self-reports, particularly for those in the nonalcoholic group, could adversely influence the sensitivity and specificity of the analysis. The issue of whether different sets of discriminant functions are needed to correctly define problem drinkers in different clinical populations needs to be investigated. This will include examination of factors such as age, sex, health or disease status, other drug intake, drinking history, and familial history of alcoholism. When new markers become available, they can be added to the conventional battery of tests to determine whether classification accuracy can be improved. The discriminant analysis of questionnaire data together with laboratory tests has been found to attain high sensitivity and specificity for excessive drinking and alcoholism (Bernadt et al., 1984). However, it should be stressed that if the same questionnaire data are used to define subject groups and in the discriminant function analysis, then the classification rates would be biased toward inflated accuracy.

## New State Markers

*Mitochondrial Aspartate Aminotransferase (MASAT).* Nalpas et al. (1984, 1986) first suggested the use of the ratio of serum MASAT/total ASAT as a highly sensitive and specific marker for chronic heavy alcohol consumption. In an *in vitro* study using hepatocytes from rats fed chronically with ethanol, Okuno et al. (1988) found an increased leakage of MASAT into the incubation medium and higher MASAT/total ASAT values than in hepatocytes from control rats. The data support the notion that MASAT can contribute to the increase in serum ASAT activity seen in alcoholics. Although the MASAT/total ASAT ratio had a high sensitivity (90 to 92%) in the classification of alcoholics (with or without liver diseases) from patients with nonalcoholic liver diseases, it had a relatively low specificity (50 to 70%) (Fletcher et al., 1991; Ink et al., 1989; Kwoh-Gain et al., 1990). The same test was also not very sensitive (0-17%, depending on cutoff limits) in distinguishing between young adult alcoholics and controls, but the specificity was high (82 to 97%, depending on cutoff limits) (Chan et al., 1989). Other recent investigations using unselected populations also showed that the MASAT test had poor sensitivity (< 30%) in detecting heavy drinking (Nalpas et al., 1989; Nilssen et al., 1992; Schiele et al., 1989).

*ß-Hexosaminidase.* The lysosomal glycosidase ß-hexosaminidase (ß-HEX) also known as N-acetyl-ß-D-glucosaminidase, has been shown to increase in alcoholics and in persons with diseases such as liver diseases, diabetes, and heart diseases (Karkkainen, 1990; Wehr et al., 1991). Several studies have reported high sensitivities (69%-94%) and specificities (> 95%) of serum ß-HEX in detecting alcoholics or heavy drinkers (Hultberg et al., 1980; Karkkainen, 1990; Karkkainen et al., 1990; Wehr et al., 1991). Urinary ß-HEX was reported to have higher sensitivity (81.3%) than serum ß-HEX (sensitivity 68.8%) in identifying alcoholics in a detoxification center (Karkkainen, 1990). The increased serum ß-HEX decreased by over 50% upon several days of abstinence (Hultberg et al., 1980; Karkkainen et al., 1990; Wehr et al., 1991), but urinary ß-HEX only decreased by about 12% after 7 days of abstinence in alcoholics (Karkkainen, 1990). Wehr et al. (1991) have shown that the increased ß-HEX activity in intoxicated alcoholics was mostly due to the thermostable component of the enzyme. Using an enzyme immunoassay Hultberg et al. (1991) analyzed the isoenzymes of ß-HEX, namely HEX A and HEX "B" (a mixture of HEX B and HEX P) in alcoholics hospitalized for detoxification and in alcoholics abstinent between 6 days and 10 years, as well as a control group. While there was considerable overlap in activity of the HEX A isoenzyme in these groups, all the hospitalized alcoholics had elevated HEX "B" isoenzyme, but only one out of the 22 abstinent patients had an increased level of HEX "B." A recent study of healthy university students by Nystrom et al. (1991) found that there was no difference in serum ß-HEX activity between the heaviest drinking group and teetotalers, and no correlation between self-reported drinking and ß-HEX activity could be demonstrated. The negative findings imply that ß-HEX may not be useful as a screening tool for heavy drinking, perhaps due to its rapid decrease upon cessation of drinking. Nevertheless, it is a potentially useful test for detecting recent excessive drinking and for monitoring of alcohol relapses in treated alcoholics. More investigations are needed to characterize the efficacy of urinary ß-HEX and HEX "B" isoenzyme in the detection of heavy drinking and/or alcoholism.

*Carbohydrate-Deficient Transferrin (CDT).* Transferrin is a glycoprotein involved in the transport and delivery of iron in the body. Since the pioneering work of Stibler (1980) showing that the serum concentration of a genetic variant of transferrin, known as carbohydrate-deficient transferrin (CDT), was increased in alcoholics and heavy drinkers, many studies (reviewed by Stibler, 1991) have confirmed that CDT has a high sensitivity (81-94%) and specificity (91-100%) as a marker for recent excessive alcohol consumption. However, some other studies (Chan et al., 1989; Chapman et al., 1985; Poupon et al., 1985, 1989) have reported relatively low sensitivity and specificity for CDT. These results were explained in terms of either technical difficulties in the analytical method or because the CDT increase in alcoholics and heavy drinkers might have been normalized because of duration of abstinence (Girela et al., 1991; Stibler, 1991). Even when these factors have been accounted for, 6-21% false-negative results for CDT have been reported (Behrens et al., 1988b; Stibler, 1991). Two recent studies, one involving the general population in a Norwegian town (Nilssen et al., 1992) and the other involving young Finnish university students (Nystrom, 1992), also reported low sensitivity (21 to 26%) but high specificity (90 to 96%) for CDT as a marker of self-reported heavy drinking. It is possible that there might have been some bingers in the heavy-drinking group who could have abstained several days before their participation in the two studies. Numerous studies have shown that CDT abnormality normalizes during abstention, with half-life of about 14 days (reviewed by Stibler, 1991). In fact, this property of CDT can be effectively utilized as a tool to assess alcoholism treatment outcome. Thus, Behrens et al. (1988b) found that the combination of CDT and GGT had a sensitivity of 95% as a marker for relapses in detoxified alcoholics. These investigators found that 80% of those alcoholics with normal CDT levels at the onset of detoxification had elevated levels of GGT which decreased progressively during abstinence. The recent commercial availability of a radioimmunoassay (RIA)-kit for CDT (Pharmacia) in the U.S. and a newly developed method for analyzing CDT (Xin et al., 1991) should facilitate further research in the use of CDT not only as a marker for recent excessive alcohol intake in other unselected populations but also as an indicator of alcoholism treatment outcome. There is also a need to explain the false-negative results found in some studies (Stibler, 1991).

*5-Hydroxytryptophol (5-HTOL).* Under normal conditions, the major urinary metabolite of serotonin is 5-hydroxyindole-3-acetic acid (5-HIAA), formed by the oxidation of 5-hydroxyindole-3-acetaldehyde and catalyzed by aldehyde dehydrogenase. Alcohol consumption induces a shift in serotonin metabolism from 5-HIAA toward formation of 5-HTOL, perhaps due to the competitive inhibition of aldehyde dehydrogenase by acetaldehyde (from metabolism of ethanol), and to increased levels of NADH during ethanol metabolism which favor 5-HTOL production (Voltaire et al., 1992). In rats an increased formation (180%) of brain 5-HTOL *in vivo* could be demonstrated at 90 minutes after an acute ethanol administration (Yoshimoto et al., 1992). The urinary ratio of 5-HTOL/5-HIAA has been proposed as a possible marker of recent alcohol consumption, with a cutoff ratio > 20. However, only a small number of subjects has been tested so far, and more research is needed to characterize this marker (including research on the influence of diet and drugs as well as responses to alcohol intake) (Voltaire et al., 1992). The potential usefulness of this test appears to be in detecting recent excessive alcohol consumption and in monitoring the effectiveness of alcoholism treatment, rather than as an indicator of alcoholism. One disadvantage is the method of analysis requires the GC/MS system.

*Acetaldehyde-Protein Adduct.* Acetaldehyde, the intermediate metabolite of ethanol oxidation, can bind to various proteins to form acetaldehyde-protein adducts (e.g., Behrens et al., 1988a; Lumeng & Durant, 1985; Tuma et al., 1987). These adducts have been demonstrated in animals fed alcohol chronically (Lin et al., 1988), in primary cultured rat hepatocytes exposed to ethanol (Lin et al., 1990a), in alcoholics (Lin et al., 1990b; Niemela et al., 1991; Wickramasinghe et al., 1989), and in social and light drinkers following an acute ethanol ingestion (Niemela et al., 1991). Different fractions of hemoglobin-acetaldehyde adducts (HbA) have been demonstrated and their potential values as markers of heavy drinking studied. Levels of the fraction HbAA correlated with scores on the Self-Administered Alcoholism Screening Test (SAAST), a useful instrument in the detection of alcoholism in medical settings (Peterson et al., 1990), but the SAAST was more sensitive than HbAA levels in the detection of alcoholics. Sillanaukee et al. (1991a,b) reported that the $HbA_{Iach}$ levels correlated with self-reports of alcohol consumption but not with levels of MCV or GGT, and that the $HbA_{Iach}/HbA_{IC}$ ratio correlated with scores of the Malmo Modified Michigan Alcoholism Screening Test (Mm-MAST). However, the sensitivity was low for these HbA fractions in the detection of heavy drinkers. The demonstration that acetaldehyde-protein adducts can act as neoantigens and the isolation of antibodies that reacted with the adducts (Israel et al., 1986, 1988; Lin et al., 1988; Worrall et al., 1989) has paved the way for antibody-based analyses of the adducts as potential markers of excessive alcohol consumption (Hoerner et al., 1988; Israel et al., 1988; Lin et al., 1990b; Niemela & Israel, 1992; Niemela et al., 1987, 1991; Worrall et al., 1990). However, the reliability of these antibodies appears to be low. For example, Niemela and Israel (1992) found that immuno-reactive HbA were increased in only 50% of alcohol abusers, but were also increased in 24% of social drinkers and 13.5% of controls. Patients with nonalcoholic liver diseases also had elevated levels of antibodies against acetaldehyde adducts (Hoerner et al., 1988; Worrall et al., 1990). A new approach using more precisely modified peptides pertaining to specific regions of hemoglobin and the generation of antibodies against them appeared to improve the sensitivity (75 to 78%) and specificity (93%) of HbA as markers of alcoholism (Lin et al., 1992). It remains to be investigated whether these improved markers are useful as screening tools for heavy drinking in unselected populations.

## CONCLUSIONS

Although there is yet no single screening instrument that has a 100% sensitivity and specificity in detecting problem drinkers and/or alcoholics in research and clinical settings, several brief and easy-to-use questionnaires reviewed in this paper can be effectively used by clinicians to screen patients for these problems. The challenge is to convince medical practitioners to routinely adopt one or more of these instruments in their clinical practices. A good starting point is the inclusion of updated information on the techniques and skills of detection of alcohol-related problems in the medical curriculum and in continuing education programs. This will also require the commitments of university administrators and professors, as well as those of hospital or clinical administrators, in the development and implementation of such programs. As one study has demonstrated, although over 90% of general practitioners felt they had a role to work with drinkers, only 40% felt capable to work with drinkers and 40% felt motivated to do so (Anderson, 1985). Armed with the necessary skills and techniques, health care professionals may be more willing to practice, and may feel less pessimistic about, effective intervention in their patients' drinking problems. Therefore, it is also necessary to convince doctors about the benefits of brief and early interventions (Anderson, 1992). There is also a need to conduct studies on the effect of a substance abuse curriculum on the recognition of heavy drinking/alcoholism by interns, residents, and professionally established doctors. This is because Susman et al. (1992) reported that despite the institution of a comprehensive substance abuse curriculum at the third year of medical studies, the history taking and correct assessment of alcohol status of family medicine residents did not improve but actually worsened with time. However, the investigators cautioned that a two-month inpatient rotation might be too short to incorporate behavioral changes in the residents' attitudes toward patients with alcohol-related problems; other limiting factors included possible inaccuracy of the measure of resident history-taking and diagnosis (i.e., chart reviews), possible burnout after a long inpatient rotation, and pessimism about effectively treating alcoholics over the short run (Susman et al., 1992).

There is a need to further validate the utility of brief screening questionnaires in unselected populations, in particular newer tests such as the TWEAK and the Cyr and Wartman (1988) two-item test. Ideally, these studies should adopt a uniform gold standard for each parameter under investigation, e.g., hazardous drinking or alcoholism. This is no easy task because of the diversity of existing definitions of terms such as heavy drinkers, alcohol abuse, alcoholism, and so on. A revised definition of alcoholism has recently been established by a panel of experts (Morse & Flavin, 1992). It is hoped that other definitions pertinent to alcohol-related problems will be agreed upon by such panels. Notwithstanding the lack of uniform gold standards, each study needs to clearly define criteria for the problems being investigated to allow for comparisons with, and replications by, other investigations. Another research area that requires attention is possible sex differences in responses to these questionnaires. It may be necessary to institute phrasing modifications or changes in cutoff scores on certain tests to accommodate such differences. As an example, gender differences in responses to the CAGE have been reported in a general population survey (Smart et al., 1991). A related issue is whether physicians are more likely to identify men who have alcoholism than women, as has been documented by Dawson et al. (1992). There also may be age differences in responses to certain screening instruments. For example, the poor sensitivity of the CAGE in a study of elderly patients (Mangion et al., 1992) may reflect the finding that most elderly alcohol abusers do not consider their drinking a problem. Another research need is to examine whether instruments such as the CAGE and B-MAST, which focus on lifetime prevalence of alcohol problems, overestimate alcohol problems in different populations. Research to date has indicated that in general questionnaire data have better sensitivity than biochemical markers in detecting problem drinkers or alcoholics. Nevertheless, there is definitely a place for biochemical markers in research as well as in clinical practice because questionnaire data are subject to inaccuracies due to poor memory recall or deliberate falsifications. An abnormal biochemical test can be effectively used by doctors to overcome a patient's denial, and to serve as a catalyst for brief intervention. Another potential advantage of biochemical markers is that they can be used to follow up on treatment effectiveness or relapses. However, more research is needed to define the optimal test or combination of tests for these purposes. Future research also needs to seek out markers for heavy binge drinking, as distinct from markers for chronic and frequent heavy drinking, and markers for heavy drinkers who have not yet developed severe physical and psychosocial problems of heavy alcohol intake.

## REFERENCES

Alterman, A. I., Gelfand, L. A., & Sweeney, K. K. (1992). The alcohol clinical index in lower socioeconomic alcohol-dependent men. *Alcoholism: Clinical and Experimental Research, 16*, 960-963.

Anderson, P. (1985). Managing alcohol problems in general practice. *British Medical Journal, 290*, 1873-1875.

Anderson, P. (1992). Primary care physicians and alcohol. *Journal of the Royal Society of Medicine, 85*, 478-482.

Babor, T. F., de la Fuente, J. R., Saunders, J., & Grant, M. (1989). AUDIT. The alcohol use disorders identification test. Guidelines for use in primary health care. *World Health Organization*, 1-24.

Baird, M. A., Burge, S. K., & Grant, W. D. (1989). A scheme for determining the prevalence of alcoholism in hospitalized patients. *Alcoholism: Clinical and Experimental Research, 13*, 782-785.

Balldin, J. I., Berggren, U. C., & Lindstedt, G. (1992). Neuroendocrine evidence for reduced dopamine receptor sensitivity in alcoholism. *Alcoholism: Clinical and Experimental Research, 16*, 71-74.

Barrett, T. G., & Williams, C. H. V. (1989). Use of a questionnaire to obtain an alcohol history from those attending an inner-city accident and emergency department. *Archives of Emergency Medicine, 6,* 34-40.

Barrison, I. G., Wright, J. T., Sampson, B., Morris, N. F., & Murray-Lyon, I. M. (1982). Screening for alcohol abuse in pregnancy. *British Medical Journal, 285,* 1318.

Begleiter, H., & Porjesz, B. (1988). Potential biological markers in individuals at high risk for developing alcoholism. *Alcoholism: Clinical and Experimental Research, 12,* 488-493.

Behrens, U. J., Hoerner, M., Lasker, J. M., & Lieber, C. S. (1988a). Formation of acetaldehyde adducts with ethanol-inducible P45OIIE1 in vivo. *Biochemical and Biophysical Research Communications, 154,* 584-590.

Behrens, U. J., Worner, T. M., & Lieber, C. S. (1988b). Changes in carbohydrate-deficient transferrin levels after alcohol withdrawal. *Alcoholism: Clinical and Experimental Research, 12,* 539-544.

Beresford, T. P., Blow, F. C., Brower, K. J., & Singer, K. (1988). Clinical applications screening for alcoholism. *Preventive Medicine, 17,* 653-663.

Beresford, T. P., Blow, F. C., Hill, E., Singer, K., & Lucey, M. R. (1990). Comparison of CAGE questionnaire and computer-assisted laboratory profiles in screening for covert alcoholism. *The Lancet, 336,* 482-485.

Bernadt, M. W., Mumford, J., & Murphy, R. M. (1984). A discriminant-function analysis of screening tests for excessive drinking and alcoholism. *Journal of Studies on Alcohol, 45,* 81-86.

Blum, K., Noble, E. P., Sheridan, P. J., Finley, O., Montgomery, A., Ritchie, T., Ozkaragoz, T., Fitch, R. J., Sadlack, F., Sheffield, D., Dahlmann, T., Halbardier, S., & Nogami, H. (1991). Association of the A1 allele of the $D_2$ dopamine receptor gene with severe alcoholism. *Alcohol, 8,* 409-416.

Blum, K., Noble, E. P., Sheridan, P. J., Montgomery, A., Ritchie, T., Jagadeeswaran, P., Nogami, H., Briggs, A. H., & Cohn, J. B. (1990). Allelic association of human dopamine $D_2$ receptor gene in alcoholism. *Journal of the American Medical Association, 263,* 2055-2060.

Bolos, A. M., Dean, M., Lucas-Derse, S., Ramsburg, M., Brown, G. L., & Goldman, D. (1990). Population and pedigree studies reveal a lack of association between the dopamine $D_2$ receptor gene and alcoholism. *Journal of the American Medical Association, 264,* 3156-3160.

Bradley, K. A. (1992). Screening and diagnosis of alcoholism in the primary care setting. *Western Journal of Medicine, 156,* 166-171.

Buchsbaum, D. G., Buchanan, R. G., Centor, R. M., Schnoll, S. H., & Lawton, M. J. (1991). Screening for alcohol abuse using CAGE scores and likelihood ratios. *Annals of Internal Medicine, 115,* 774-777.

Bush, B., Shaw, S., Cleary, P., Delbanco, T. L., & Aronson, M. D. (1987). Screening for alcohol abuse using the CAGE questionnaire. *The American Journal of Medicine, 82,* 231-235.

Chan, A. W. K. (1990). Biochemical markers for alcoholism. In M. Windle & J. S. Searles (Eds.), *Children of alcoholics: Critical perspectives,* (pp. 39-71). New York: The Guilford Press.

Chan, A. W. K. (1991). Multiple drug use in drug and alcohol addiction. In N. S. Miller (Ed.), *Comprehensive handbook of drug and alcohol addiction*, (pp. 87-113). White Plain, NY: Marcel Dekker, Inc.

Chan, A. W. K., Leong, F. W., Schanley, D. L., Welte, J. W., Wieczorek, W., Rej, R., & Whitney, R. B. (1989). Transferrin and mitochondrial aspartate aminotransferase in young adult alcoholics. *Drug and Alcohol Dependence, 23,* 13-18.

Chang, M. M., Kwon, J., Hamada, R. S., & Yahiku, P. (1990). Effect of combined substance use on laboratory markers of alcoholism. *Journal of Studies on Alcohol, 51,* 361-365.

Chapman, R. W., Sorrentino, D., & Morgan, M. Y. (1985). Abnormal heterogeneity of serum transferrin in relation to alcohol consumption: A reappraisal. In N. C. Chang & H. M. Chao (Eds.), *NIAAA Research Monograph 17 Early identification of alcohol abuse,* (pp. 108-114). Rockville, MD: U.S. Department of Health and Human Services.

Chick, J., Kreitman, N., & Plant, M. (1981). Mean cell volume and gamma-glutamyl transpeptidase as markers of drinking in working men. *Lancet, 1,* 1249-1251.

Ciraulo, D. A., Barnhill, J. G., Ciraulo, A. M., Greenblatt, D. J., & Shader, R. I. (1989). Parental alcoholism as a risk factor in benzodiazepine abuse: A pilot study. *American Journal of Psychiatry, 146,* 1333-1335.

Cloninger, C. R. (1991). D2 dopamine receptor gene is associated but not linked with alcoholism. *Journal of the American Medical Association, 266,* 1833-1834.

Comings, D. E., Comings, B. G., Muhleman, D., Dietz, G., Shahbahrami, B., Tast, D., Knell, E., Kocsis, P., Baumgarten, R., Kovacs, B. W., Levy, D. L., Smith, M., Borison, R. L., Evans, D. D., Klein, D. N., MacMurray, J., Tosk, J. M., Sverd, J., Gysin, R., & Flanagan, S. D. (1991). The dopamine D2 receptor locus as a modifying gene in neuropsychiatric disorders. *Journal of the American Medical Association, 266,* 1793-1800.

Conigrave, K. M., Burns, F. H., Reznik, R. B., & Saunders, J. B. (1991). Problem drinking in emergency department patients: The scope for early intervention. *Medical Journal of Australia, 154,* 801-805.

Cook, B. L., Wang, Z. W., Crowe, R. R., Hauser, R., & Freimer, M. (1992). Alcoholism and the D2 receptor gene. *Alcoholism: Clinical and Experimental Research, 16,* 806-809.

Crabb, D. W. (1990). Biological markers for increased risk of alcoholism and for quantitation of alcohol consumption. *Journal of Clinical Investigation, 85,* 311-315.

Cushman, P., Jacobson, G., Barboriak, J. J., & Anderson, A. J. (1984). Biochemical markers for alcoholism: Sensitivity problems. *Alcoholism: Clinical and Experimental Research, 8,* 253-257.

Cyr, M. G., & Wartman, S. A. (1988). The effectiveness of routine screening questions in the detection of alcoholism. *Journal of the American Medical Association, 259,* 51-54.

Dawson, N. V., Dadheech, G., Speroff, T., Smith, R.L., & Schubert D. S. P. (1992). The effect of patient gender on the prevalence and recognition of alcoholism on a general medicine inpatient service. *Journal of General Internal Medicine, 7*, 38-45.

Devor, E. J., & Cloninger, C. R. (1989). Genetics of alcoholism. *Annual Review of Genetics, 23*, 19-36.

Devor, E. J., Cloninger, C. R., Hoffman, P. L., & Tabakoff, B. (1991). A genetic study of platelet adenylate cyclase activity: Evidence for a single major locus effect in fluoride-stimulated activity. *American Journal of Human Genetics, 49*, 372-377.

De Wit, H. (1991). Diazepam preference in males with and without an alcoholic first-degree relative. *Alcoholism: Clinical and Experimental Research, 15*, 593-600.

De Wit, H., & McCracken, S. G. (1990). Ethanol self-administration in males with and without an alcoholic first-degree relative. *Alcoholism: Clinical and Experimental Research, 14*, 63-70.

Diamond, I., Wrubel, B., Estrin, W., & Gordon, A. (1987). Basal and adenosine receptor-stimulated levels of cyclic AMP are reduced in lymphocytes from alcoholic patients. *Proceedings of the National Academy of Science. U. S. A. 84*, 1413-1416.

Dobkin, P., Dongier, M., Cooper, D., & Hill, J. M. (1991). Screening for alcoholism in a psychiatric hospital. *Canadian Journal of Psychiatry, 36*, 39-45.

Eckardt, M. J., Rawlings, R. R., & Martin, P. R. (1986). Biological correlates and detection of alcohol abuse and alcoholism. *Progress in Neuro-Psychopharmacology & Biological Psychiatry, 10*, 135-144.

Engs, R. C. (1990). Family background of alcohol abuse and its relationship to alcohol consumption among college students: An unexpected finding. *Journal of Studies on Alcohol, 51*, 542-547.

Eskay, R., & Linnoila, M. (1991). Potential biochemical markers for the predisposition toward alcoholism. In M. Galanter (Ed.), *Recent development in alcoholism*, (Vol. 9) (pp. 41-51). New York: Plenum Press.

Ewing, J. A. (1984). Detecting alcoholism. The CAGE questionnaire. *Journal of the American Medical Association, 252*, 1905-1907.

Fleming, M. F., Barry, K. L., & MacDonald, R. (1991). The alcohol use disorders identification test (AUDIT) in a college sample. *The International Journal of the Addictions, 26*, 1173-1185.

Fletcher, L. M., Kwoh-Gain, I., Powell, E. E., Powell, L. W., & Halliday, J. W. (1991). Markers of chronic alcohol ingestion in patients with nonalcoholic steatohepatitis: An aid to diagnosis. *Hepatology, 13*, 455-459.

Gelernter, J., O'Malley, S., Risch, N., Kranzler, H. R., Krystal, J., Merikangas, K., Kennedy, J. L., & Kidd, K. K. (1991). No association between an allele at the $D_2$ dopamine receptor gene (DRD2) and alcoholism. *Journal of the American Medical Association, 266*, 1801-1807.

German, E. (1973). Medical problems in chronic alcoholic men. *Journal of Chronic Diseases, 26*, 661-668.

Girela, E., Hernandez-Cueto, C., & Villanueva, E. (1991). Carbohydrate-deficient transferrin (CDT) as indicator of alcohol misuse: Evaluation of problems in the methodology. *Alcohol & Alcoholism, 26,* 653-654.

Goldberg, H. I., Mullen, M., Ries, R. K., Psaty, B. M., & Ruch, B. P. (1991). Alcohol counseling in a general medicine clinic. *Medical Care, 29,* 49-56.

Gordis, E., Tabakoff, B., Goldman, D., & Berg, K. (1990). Finding the gene(s) for alcoholism. *Journal of the American Medical Association, 263,* 2094-2095.

Graham, A. W. (1991). Screening for alcoholism by life-style risk assessment in a community hospital. *Archives of Internal Medicine, 151,* 958-964.

Halmesmaki, E., Roine, R., & Salaspuro, M. (1992). Gamma-glutamyltransferase, aspartate and alanine aminotransferases and their ratio, mean cell volume and urinary dolichol in pregnant alcohol abusers. *British Journal of Obstetrics and Gynaecology, 99,* 287-291.

Heck, E. J., & Lichtenberg, J. W. (1990). Validity of the CAGE in screening for problem drinking in college students. *Journal of College Student Development, 31,* 359-364.

Hill, S. Y., Aston, C., & Robin, B. (1988). Suggestive evidence of genetic linkage between alcoholism and the MNS blood group. *Alcoholism: Clinical and Experimental Research, 12,* 811-814.

Hill, S. Y., Steinhauer, S. R., & Zubin, J. (1987). Biological markers for alcoholism: A vulnerability model conceptualization. In P. C. Rivers (Ed.), *Alcohol and addictive behavior: Nebraska symposium on motivation,* (pp. 207-256). Lincoln: University of Nebraska Press.

Hill, S. Y., Zubenko, G. S., Gronlund, S., & Teply, I. (1991). Ethanol's fluidizing effects on RBC membranes from children at risk for alcoholism. *Alcohol, 8,* 405-407.

Hiller, W., Mombour, W., & Mittelhammer, J. (1989). A systematic evaluation of the DSM-III-R criteria for alcohol dependence. *Comprehensive Psychiatry, 30,* 403-415.

Hoerner, M., Behrens, U. J., Worner, T. M., Blacksberg, I., Braly, L. F., Schaffner, F., & Lieber, C. S. (1988). The role of alcoholism and liver disease in the appearance of serum antibodies against acetaldehyde adducts. *Hepatology, 8,* 569-574.

Holt, S., Skinner, H. A., & Israel, Y. (1981). Early identification of alcohol abuse: 2: Clinical and laboratory indicators. *Canadian Medical Association Journal, 124,* 1279-1295.

Hultberg, B., Isaksson, A., Berglund, M., & Moberg, A. L. (1991). Serum beta-hexosaminidase isoenzyme: A sensitive marker for alcohol abuse. *Alcoholism: Clinical and Experimental Research, 15,* 549-552.

Hultberg, B., Isaksson, A., & Tiderstrom, G. (1980). ß-hexosaminidase, leucine aminopeptidase, hepatic enzymes and bilirubin in serum of chronic alcoholics with acute ethanol intoxication. *Clinica Chimica Acta, 105,* 317-323.

Ink, O., Boutron, A., Hanny, P., Goenner, S., & Buffet, C. (1989). Serum mitochondrial aspartate aminotransferase activity as marker of alcohol intoxication in cirrhotic patients. *Presse Medicale, 18,* 111-114.

Israel, Y., Hurwitz, E., Niemela, O., & Arnon, R. (1986). Monoclonal and polyclonal antibodies against acetaldehyde-containing epitopes in acetaldehyde-protein adducts. *Proceedings of the National Academy of Science of the United States of America, 83,* 7923-7927.

Israel, Y., Orrego, H., & Niemela, O. (1988). Immune responses to alcohol metabolites: Pathogenic and diagnostic implications. *Seminars in Liver Disease, 8,* 81-90.

Karkkainen, P. (1990). Serum and urinary beta-hexosaminidase as markers of heavy drinking. *Alcohol & Alcoholism, 25,* 365-369.

Karkkainen, P., Poikolainen, K., & Salaspuro, M. (1990). Serum ß-hexosaminidase as a marker of heavy drinking. *Alcoholism: Clinical and Experimental Research, 14,* 187-190.

Katerer, R. M. H., Carulli, N., & Iber, F. L. (1969). Differences in the rate of ethanol metabolism, in recently drinking alcoholic and nondrinking subjects. *American Journal of Clinical Nutrition, 22,* 1608-1617.

Kent, A. (1991). Measure of alcohol dependence. *The Lancet, 338,* 889.

Keso, L., & Salaspuro, M. (1990a). Comparative value of self-report and blood tests in assessing outcome amongst alcoholics. *British Journal of Addiction, 85,* 209-215.

Keso, L., & Salaspuro, M. (1990b). Laboratory tests in the follow-up of treated alcoholics: How often should testing be repeated? *Alcohol & Alcoholism, 25,* 359-363.

Klatsky, A. L., Friedman, G. D., & Siegelaub, A. B. (1981). Alcohol and mortality: a ten-year Kaiser Permanente experience. *Annals of Internal Medicine, 95,* 139-145.

Kolb, D., & Gunderson, E. (1983). Medical histories of problem drinkers during their first twelve years of naval service. *Journal of Studies on Alcohol, 44,* 84-94.

Kristenson, H., & Trell, E. (1982). Indicators of alcohol consumption: comparisons between a questionnaire (MmMAST), interviews and serum-gamma glutamyltransferase (GGT) in a health survey of middle-aged males. *British Journal of Addiction, 77,* 297-304.

Kwoh-Gain, I., Fletcher, L. M., Price J., Powell, L. W., & Halliday, J. W. (1990). Desialylated transferrin and mitochondrial aspartate aminotransferase compared as laboratory markers of excessive alcohol consumption. *Clinical Chemistry, 36,* 841-845.

Latcham, R. W. (1986). Gamma-glutamyl transpeptidase and mean corpuscular volume: Their usefulness in the assessment of in-patient alcoholics. *British Journal of Psychiatry, 149,* 353-356.

Levenson, R. W., Oyama, O. N., & Meek, P. S. (1987). Greater reinforcement from alcohol for those at risk: Parental risk, personality risk, and sex. *Journal of Abnormal Psychology, 96,* 242-253.

Lex, B. W., Ellingboe, J. E., Teoh, S. K., Mendelson, J. H., & Rhoades, E. (1991). Prolactin and cortisol levels following acute alcohol challenges in women with and without a family history of alcoholism. *Alcohol, 8,* 383-387.

Lin, R. C., Fillenwarth, M. J., Minter, R., & Lumeng, L. (1990a). Formation of the 37-KD protein-acetaldehyde adduct in primary cultured rat hepatocytes exposed to alcohol. *Hepatology, 11*, 401-407.

Lin, R. C., Lumeng, L., Shahidi, S., Kelly, T., & Pound, D. C. (1990b). Protein-acetaldehyde adducts in serum of alcoholic patients. *Alcoholism: Clinical and Experimental Research, 14*, 438-443.

Lin, R. C., Shahidi, S., Kelly, T. J., Lumeng, C., & Lumeng, L. (1992). Measurement of hemoglobin-acetaldehyde adducts (Hb-AA) in alcoholic patients. *Alcohol and Alcoholism, 27*, (supplement 1), 81.

Lin, R. C., Smith, R. S., & Lumeng, L. (1988). Detection of a protein-acetaldehyde adduct in the liver of rats fed alcohol chronically. *Journal of Clinical Investigation, 81*, 615-619.

Loosen, P. T., Marciniak, R., & Thadani, K. (1987). TRH-induced TSH response in healthy volunteers: Relationship to psychiatric history. *American Journal of Psychiatry, 144*, 455-459.

Lumeng, L. (1986). New diagnostic markers of alcohol abuse. *Hepatology, 6*, 742-745.

Lumeng, L., & Durant, P. J. (1985). Regulation of the formation of stable adducts between acetaldehyde and blood proteins. *Alcohol, 2*, 397-400.

Mangion, D. M., Platt, J., & Syam, V. (1992). Alcohol and acute medical admission of elderly people. *Age and Ageing, 21*, 362-367.

Mayfield, D., McLeod, G., & Hall, P. (1974). The CAGE questionnaire: Validation of a new alcoholism screening instrument. *American Journal of Psychiatry, 131*, 1121-1123.

McCaul, M. E., Turkkan, J. S., Svikis, D. S., & Bigelow, G. E. (1990). Alcohol and secobarbital effects as a function of familial alcoholism: Acute psychophysiological effects. *Alcoholism: Clinical and Experimental Research, 14*, 704-712.

McCaul, M. E., Turkkan, J. S., Svikis, D. S., & Bigelow, G. E. (1991). Alcohol and secobarbital effects as a function of familial alcoholism: Extended intoxication and increased withdrawal effects. *Alcoholism: Clinical and Experimental Research, 15*, 94-101.

Mihas, A. T., & Tavassoli, M. (1992). Laboratory markers of ethanol intake and abuse: A critical appraisal. *American Journal of Medical Sciences, 303*, 415-428.

Mischke, H. D., & Venneri, R. L. (1987). Reliability and validity of the MAST, Mortimer-Filkins Questionnaire and CAGE in DWI assessment. *Journal of Studies on Alcohol, 48*, 492-501.

Monteiro, M. G., Irwin, M., Hauger, R. L., & Schuckit, M. A. (1990). TSH response to TRH and family history of alcoholism. *Biological Psychiatry, 27*, 905-910.

Moore, R. D., Bone, L. R., Geller, G., Mamon, J. A., Stokes, E. J., & Levine, D. M. (1989). Prevalence, detection, and treatment of alcoholism in hospitalized patients. *The Journal of the American Medical Association, 261*, 403-407.

Moran, M. B., Naughton, B. J., & Hughes, S. L. (1990). Screening elderly veterans for alcoholism. *Journal of General Internal Medicine, 5*, 361-364.

Morse, R. M., & Flavin, D. K. (1992). The definition of alcoholism. *Journal of the American Medical Association, 268*, 1012-1014.

Moss, H. B., Yao, J. K., Burns, M., Maddock, J., & Tarter, R. E. (1990). Plasma GABA-like activity in response to ethanol challenge in men at high risk for alcoholism. *Biological Psychiatry, 27*, 617-625.

Moss, H. B., Yao, J. K., & Maddock, J. (1989). Responses by sons of alcoholic fathers to alcoholic and placebo drinks: Perceived mood, intoxication and plasma prolactin. *Alcoholism: Clinical and Experimental Research, 13*, 252-257.

Nalpas, B., Poupon, R. E., Vassault A., Hauzanneau, P., Sage, Y., Schellenberg, F., Lacour, B., & Berthelot, P. (1989). Evaluation of mMAST/tTAST ratio as a marker of alcohol misuse in a nonselected population. *Alcohol & Alcoholism, 24*, 415-419.

Nalpas, B., Vassault, A., Charpin, S., Lacour, B., & Berthelot, P. (1986). Serum mitochondrial aspartate aminotransferase as a marker of chronic alcoholism: Diagnostic value and interpretation in a liver unit. *Hepatology, 6*, 608-614.

Nalpas, B., Vassault, A., Guillou, A. L., Lesgourgues, B., Ferry, N., Lacour, B., & Berthelot, P. (1984). Serum activity of mitochondrial aspartate aminotransferase: A sensitive marker of alcoholism with or without alcoholic hepatitis. *Hepatology, 4*, 893-896.

National Council on Alcoholism, Criteria Committee (1972). Criteria for the diagnosis of alcoholism. *American Journal of Psychiatry, 129*, 127-135.

Newlin, D. B., & Pretorius, M. B. (1990). Sons of alcoholics report greater hangover symptoms than sons of nonalcoholics: A pilot study. *Alcoholism: Clinical and Experimental Research, 14*, 713-716.

Newlin, D. B., & Thomson, J. B. (1991). Chronic tolerance and sensitization to alcohol in sons of alcoholics. *Alcoholism: Clinical and Experimental Research, 15*, 399-405.

Niemela, O., & Israel, Y. (1992). Hemoglobin-acetaldehyde adducts in human alcohol abusers. *Laboratory Investigation, 67*, 246-252.

Niemela, O., Juvonen, T., & Parkkila, S. (1991). Immunohistochemical demonstration of acetaldehyde-modified epitopes in human liver after alcohol consumption. *Journal of Clinical Investigation, 87*, 1367-1374.

Niemela, O., Klajner, F., Orrego, H., Vidins, E., Blendis, L., & Israel, Y. (1987). Antibodies against acetaldehyde-modified protein epitopes in human alcoholics. *Hepatology, 7*, 1210-1214.

Nilssen, O., Huseby, N. E., Hoyer, G., Brenn, T., Schirmer, H., & Forde, O. H. (1992). New alcohol markers–How useful are they in population studies: The Svalbard study 1988-89. *Alcoholism: Clinical and Experimental Research, 16*, 82-86.

Noble, E. P., Blum, K., Ritchie, T., Montgomery, A., & Sheridan, P. J. (1991). Allelic association of the D$_2$ dopamine receptor gene with receptor-binding characteristics in alcoholism. *Archives of General Psychiatry, 48*, 648-654.

Nystrom, M., Perasalo, J., & Salaspuro, M. (1991). Serum beta-hexosaminidase in young university students. *Alcoholism: Clinical and Experimental Research, 15*, 877-880.

Nystrom, M., Perasalo, J., & Salaspuro, M. (1992). Carbohydrate-deficient transferrin (CDT) in serum as a possible indicator of heavy drinking in young university students. *Alcoholism: Clinical and Experimental Research, 16*, 93-97.

Okuno, F., Ishii, H., Kashiwazaki, K., Takagi, S., Shigeta, Y., Arai, M., Takagi, T., Ebihara, Y., & Tsuchiya, M. (1988). Increase in mitochondrial GOT (m-GOT) activity after chronic alcohol consumption: Clinical and experimental observations. *Alcohol, 5*, 49-53.

Olsen, H., Sakshaug, J., Duckert, F., Stromme, J. H., & Morland, J. (1989). Ethanol elimination-rates determined by breath analysis as a marker of recent excessive ethanol consumption. *Scandinavian Journal of Clinical and Laboratory Investigation, 49*, 359-365.

O'Malley, S. S., & Maisto, S. A. (1985). The effects of family drinking history on responses to alcohol: Expectancies and reactions to intoxication. *Journal of Studies on Alcohol, 46*, 289-297.

Orrego, H., Blake, J. E., & Israel, Y. (1985). Relationship between gamma-glutamyl transpeptidase and mean urinary alcohol levels in alcoholics while drinking and after alcohol withdrawal. *Alcoholism: Clinical and Experimental Research, 9*, 10-13.

Parsian, A., Todd, R. D., Devor, E. J., O'Malley, K. L., Suarez, B. K., Reich, T., & Cloninger, C. R. (1991). Alcoholism and alleles of the human $D_2$ dopamine receptor locus. *Archives of General Psychiatry, 48*, 655-663.

Peterson, C. M., Ross, S. L., & Scott, B. K. (1990). Correlation of self-administered alcoholism screening test with hemoglobin-associated acetaldehyde. *Alcohol, 7*, 289-293.

Pileire, B., Brendent-Bangou, J., & Valentino, M. (1991). Comparison of questionnaire and biochemical markers to detect alcohol abuse in a West Indian population. *Alcohol & Alcoholism, 26*, 353-359.

Pokorny, A. D., Miller, B. A., & Kaplan, H. B. (1972). The brief MAST: a shortened version of the Michigan Alcoholism Screening Test. *American Journal of Psychiatry, 129*, 118-121.

Pollock, V. E., Teasdale, T. W., Garielli, W. F., & Knop, J. (1986). Subjective and objective measures of response to alcohol among young men at risk for alcoholism. *Journal of Studies on Alcohol, 47*, 297-304.

Poupon, R. E., Papoz, L., Sarmini, H., & Elinck, R. (1985). A study of the microheterogeneity of transferrin in cirrhotic patients. *Clinica Chimica Acta, 151*, 245-251.

Poupon, R. E., Schellenberg, F., Nalpas, B., & Weill. J. (1989). Assessment of the transferrin index in screening heavy drinkers from a general practice. *Alcoholism: Clinical and Experimental Research, 13*, 549-553.

Rausch, J. L., Monteiro, M. G., & Schuckit, M. A. (1991). Platelet serotonin uptake in men with family histories of alcoholism. *Neuropsychopharmacology,* *4,* 83-86.

Rosman, A. S., & Lieber, C. S. (1990). Biochemical markers of alcohol consumption. *Alcohol Health & Research World, 14,* 210-218.

Russell, M., Martier, S. S., Sokol, R. J., Jacobson, S., Jacobson, J., & Bottoms, S. (1991). Screening for pregnancy risk-drinking: Tweaking the tests. *Alcoholism: Clinical and Experimental Research, 15,* 368.

Ryback, R. S., Eckardt, M. J., & Pautler, C. P. (1980). Biochemical and hematological correlates of alcoholism. *Research Communications in Chemical Pathology and Pharmacology, 27,* 533-550.

Ryback, R. S., Eckardt, M. J., Rawlings, R. R., & Rosenthal, L. S. (1982). Quadratic discriminant analysis as an aid to interpretive reporting of clinical laboratory tests. *Journal of the American Medical Association, 248,* 2342-2345.

Rydon, P., Redman, S., Sanson-Fisher, R. W., & Reid, A. L. A. (1992). Detection of alcohol-related problems in general practice. *Journal of Studies on Alcohol, 53,* 197-202.

Salaspuro, M. (1986). Conventional and coming laboratory markers of alcoholism and heavy drinking. *Alcoholism: Clinical and Experimental Research, 10,* 5S-12S.

Saunders, J. B., & Foulds, K. (1992). Brief and early intervention: Experience from studies of harmful drinking. *Australian and New Zealand Journal of Medicine, 22,* 224-230.

Schiele, F., Artur, Y., Varasteh, A., Wellman, M., & Siest, G. (1989). Serum mitochondrial aspartate aminotransferase activity: Not useful as a marker of excessive alcohol consumption in an unselected population. *Clinical Chemistry, 35,* 926-930.

Schuckit, M. (1980). Self-rating of alcohol intoxication by young men with and without family histories of alcoholism. *Journal of Studies on Alcohol, 41,* 242-249.

Schuckit, M. A. (1984). Subjective responses to alcohol in sons of alcoholics and control subjects. *Archives of General Psychiatry, 41,* 879-884.

Schuckit, M. A. (1986). Biological markers in alcoholism. *Progress in Neuro-Psychopharmacology and Biological Psychiatry, 10,* 191-199.

Schuckit, M. A. (1987). Why don't we diagnose alcoholism in our patients. *The Journal of Family Practice, 25,* 225-226.

Schuckit, M. A. (1992). Advances in understanding the vulnerability to alcoholism. In C. P. O'Brien & J. H. Jaffe (Eds.), *Addictive states,* (pp. 93-108). New York: Raven Press, Ltd.

Schuckit, M. A., Duthie, L. A., Mahler, H. I. M., Irwin, M., & Monteiro, M. G. (1991a). Subjective feelings and changes in body sway following diazepam in sons of alcoholics and control subjects. *Journal of Studies on Alcohol, 52,* 601-608.

Schuckit, M. A., Gold, E., & Risch, C. (1987a). Plasma cortisol levels following ethanol in sons of alcoholics and controls. *Archives of General Psychiatry, 44,* 942-945.

Schuckit, M. A., Gold, E., & Risch, C. (1987b). Serum prolactin levels in sons of alcoholics and control subjects. *American Journal of Psychiatry, 144*, 854-859.

Schuckit, M. A., Hauger, R. L., Monteiro, M. G., Irwin, M., Duthie, L. A., & Mahler, H. I. M. (1991b). Response of three hormones to diazepam challenge in sons of alcoholics and controls. *Alcoholism: Clinical and Experimental Research, 15*, 537-542.

Schuckit, M. A., & Irwin, M. (1988). Diagnosis of alcoholism. *Medical Clinics of North America, 72*, 1133-1153.

Scott, E., & Anderson, P. (1990). Randomized controlled trial of general practitioner intervention in women with excessive alcohol consumption. *Drug and Alcohol Review, 10*, 313-321.

Selzer, M. L. (1971). The Michigan Alcoholism Screening Test: The quest for a new diagnostic instrument. *American Journal of Psychiatry, 127*, 89-94.

Selzer, M. L., Vinokur, A., & Van Roouen, L. (1975). A self-administered short Michigan Alcoholism Screening Test (SMAST). *Journal of Studies on Alcohol, 36*, 117-126.

Seppa, K., Sillanaukee, P., & Koivula, T. (1992). Abnormalities of hematologic parameters in heavy drinkers and alcoholics. *Alcoholism: Clinical and Experimental Research, 16*, 117-121.

Sillanaukee, P., Seppa, K., & Koivula, T. (1991a). Effect of acetaldehyde on hemoglobin: $HbA_{1ach}$ as a potential marker of heavy drinking. *Alcohol, 8*, 377-381.

Sillanaukee, P., Seppa, K., & Koivula, T. (1991b). Association of a haemoglobin-acetaldehyde adduct with questionnaire results on heavy drinkers. *Alcohol & Alcoholism, 26*, 519-525.

Skinner, H. A., & Holt, S. (1987). *The alcohol clinical index: Strategies for identifying patients with alcohol problems.* Toronto: Alcoholism and Drug Addiction Research Foundation.

Skinner, H. A., Holt, S., Sheu, W. J., & Israel, Y. (1986). Clinical versus laboratory detection of alcohol abuse: The alcohol clinical index. *British Medical Journal, 292*, 1703-1708.

Smart, R., Adlaf, E. M., & Knoke, D. (1991). Use of the CAGE scale in a population survey of drinking. *Journal of Studies on Alcohol, 52*, 593-596.

Smith, G.S., & Kraus, J.F. (1988). Alcohol and residential, recreational, and occupational injuries: A review of the epidemiologic evidence. *Annual Review of Public Health, 9*, 99-121.

Sokol, R. J., Martier, S. S., & Ager, J. W. (1989). The T-ACE questions: Practical prenatal detection of risk-drinking. *American Journal of Obstetrics and Gynecology, 160*, 863-870.

Stibler, H. (1991). Carbohydrate-deficient transferrin in serum: A new marker of potentially harmful alcohol consumption reviewed. *Clinical Chemistry, 37*, 2029-2037.

Stibler, H., Borg, S., & Allgulander, C. (1980). Abnormal microheterogeneity of transferrin: A new marker of alcoholism. *Substance and Alcohol Actions/Misuse, 1*, 247-252.

Susman, J., Sitorius, M., Schneider, M., & Gilbert, C. (1992). Effect of a substance abuse curriculum on the recognition of alcoholism by family medicine residents. *Journal of Alcohol and Drug Education, 38*, 98-105.

Swenson, W. M., & Morse, R. M. (1975). The use of a self-administered alcoholism screening test (SAAST) in a medical center. *Mayo Clinic Proceedings, 50*, 204-208.

Tabakoff, B., & Hoffman, P. L. (1988). Genetics and biological markers of risk for alcoholism. *Public Health Reports, 103*, 690-698.

Tabakoff, B., Hoffman, P. L., Lee, J. M., Saito, T., Willard, B., & De Leon-Jones, F. (1988). Differences in platelet enzyme activity between alcoholics and nonalcoholics. *The New England Journal of Medicine, 318*, 1134-1139.

Tang, B. K. (1987). Detection of ethanol in urine of abstaining alcoholics. *Canadian Journal of Physiology and Pharmacology, 65*, 1225-1227.

Tang, B. K. (1991). Urinary markers of chronic excessive ethanol consumption. *Alcoholism: Clinical and Experimental Research, 15*, 881-885.

Tang, B. K., Devenyi, P., Teller, D., & Israel, Y. (1986). Detection of an alcohol-specific product in urine of alcoholics. *Biochemical and Biophysical Research Communications, 140*, 924-927.

Tanna, V. L., Wilson, A. F., Winokur, G., & Elston, R. C. (1988). Possible linkage between alcoholism and esterase-D. *Journal of Studies on Alcohol, 49*, 472-476.

Tarter, R. E., Laird, S. B., & Moss, H. B. (1990). Neuropsychological and neurophysiological characteristics of children of alcoholics. In M. Windle & J. S. Searles (Eds.), *Children of alcoholics: Critical perspectives*, (pp. 73-98). New York: The Guilford Press.

Teoh, S. K., Lex, B. W., Mendelson, J. H., Mello, N. K., & Cochin, J. (1992). Hyperprolactinemia and macrocytosis in women with alcohol and polysubstance dependence. *Journal of Studies on Alcohol, 53*, 176-182.

Tuma, D. J., Jennett, R. B., & Sorrell, M. F. (1987). The interaction of acetaldehyde with tubulin. *Annals of the New York Academy of Sciences, 492*, 277-286.

Turner, E., Ewing, J., Shilling, P., Smith, T. L., Irwin, M., Schuckit, M., and Kelsoe, J. R. (1992). Lack of association between an RFLP near the $D_2$ dopamine receptor gene and severe alcoholism. *Biological Psychiatry, 31*, 285-290.

Ugarte, G., Iturriaga, H., & Pereda, T. (1977). Possible relationship between the rate of ethanol metabolism and the severity of hepatic damage in chronic alcoholics. *Digestive Diseases, 22*, 406-410.

Uhl, G. R., Persico, A. M., & Smith, S. S. (1992). Current excitement with $D_2$ dopamine receptor gene alleles in substance abuse. *Archives of General Psychiatry, 49*, 157-160.

Umbricht-Schneiter, A., Santora, P., & Moore, R. D. (1991). Alcohol abuse. Comparison of two methods for assessing its prevalence and associated morbidity in hospitalized patients. *The American Journal of Medicine, 91*, 110-118.

Vanclay, F., Raphael, B., Dunne, M., Whitfield, J., Lewin, T., & Singh, B. (1991). A community screening test for high alcohol consumption using biochemical and hematological measures. *Alcohol & Alcoholism, 26*, 337-346.

Vogel-Sprott, M., & Chipperfield, B. (1987). Family history of problem drinking among male social drinkers: Behavioral effects of alcohol. *Journal of Studies on Alcohol, 48,* 430-436.

Voltaire, A., Beck, O., & Borg, S. (1992). Urinary 5-hydroxytryptophol: A possible marker of recent alcohol consumption. *Alcoholism: Clinical and Experimental Research, 16,* 281-285.

Wallace, P., Cutler, S., & Haines, A. (1988). Randomised controlled trial of general practitioner intervention in patients with excessive alcohol consumption. *British Medical Journal, 297,* 663-668.

Watson, R. R., Mohs, M. E., Eskelson, C., Sampliner, R. E., & Hartmann, B. (1986). Identification of alcohol abuse and alcoholism with biological parameters. *Alcoholism: Clinical and Experimental Research, 10,* 364-385.

Wehr, H., Czartoryska, B., Gorska, D., & Matsumoto, H. (1991). Serum ß-hexosaminidase and alpha-mannosidase activities as markers of alcohol abuse. *Alcoholism: Clinical and Experimental Research, 15,* 13-15.

Whipple, S. C., Berman, S. M., & Noble, E. P. (1991). Event-related potentials in alcoholic fathers and their sons. *Alcohol, 8,* 321-327.

Wickramasinghe, S. N., Marjot, D. H., Rosalki, S. B., & Fink, R. S. (1989). Correlations between serum proteins modified by acetaldehyde and biochemical variables in heavy drinkers. *Journal of Clinical Pathology, 42,* 295-299.

Wieczorek, W. F., Miller, B. A., & Nochajski, T. H. (1992). The limited utility of BAC for identifying alcohol-related problems among DWI offenders. *Journal of Studies on Alcohol, 53,* 415-419.

Wilson, J. R., & Nagoshi, C. T. (1988). Adult children of alcoholics: Cognitive and psychomotor characteristics. *British Journal of Addiction, 83,* 809-820.

Worobec, T. G., Turner, W. M., O'Farrell, T. J., Cutter, H. S., Bayog, R. D., & Tsuang, M. T. (1990). Alcohol use by alcoholics with and without a history of parental alcoholism. *Alcoholism: Clinical and Experimental Research, 14,* 887-892.

Worrall, S., DeJersey, J., Shanley, B. C., & Wilce, P. A. (1990). Antibodies against acetaldehyde-modified epitopes: Presence in alcoholic, nonalcoholic liver disease and control subjects. *Alcohol & Alcoholism, 25,* 509-517.

Worrall, S., DeJersey, J., Shanley, B. C., & Wilce, P. A. (1989). Ethanol induces the production of antibodies to acetaldehyde-modified epitopes in rats. *Alcohol & Alcoholism, 24,* 217-223.

Xin, Y., Lasker, J. M., Rosman, A. S., & Lieber, C. S. (1991). Isoelectric focusing/western blotting: A novel and practical method for quantitation of carbohydrate-deficient transferrin in alcoholics. *Alcoholism: Clinical and Experimental Research, 15,* 814-821.

Ylikorkala, O., Stenman, U. H., & Halmesmaki, E. (1987). Gamma-glutamyl transferase and mean cell volume reveal maternal alcohol abuse and fetal alcohol effects. *American Journal of Obstetrics and Gynecology, 157,* 344-348.

Yoshimoto, K., Komura, S., & Kawamura, K. (1992). Occurrence in vivo of 5-hydroxytryptophol in the brain of rats treated with ethanol. *Alcohol & Alcoholism, 27,* 131-136.

# Modern Disease Models of Alcoholism and Other Chemical Dependencies: The New Biopsychosocial Models

## John Wallace

SUMMARY. A considerable body of research has indicated that alcoholism and other chemical dependencies are multidimensional phenomena. Biological, psychological, and sociocultural variables enter into the origins, nature, maintenance, and change of these disorders. Hence, continued debate and argument over the "correct" unidimensional model is unlikely to prove fruitful. Neither a naive disease concept nor a naive behavioral concept can explain addictive disorders fully. Multidimensional, interactive, biopsychosocial models are now necessary for continued progress in understanding and altering these disorders and the many personal and societal problems associated with them.

It is difficult to identify a concept that has had greater impact on the chemical dependence field than the traditional disease concept of alcoholism. The notion that chemically dependent people suffer from illnesses permitted important societal and personal responses to these problems that were not likely under other mind sets. Widespread acceptance of the traditional disease concept of alcoholism served to reduce the stigma associated with the problem, helped

John Wallace is President of AGAPE House. Address correspondence to Center for Music and Literature, 7 Clinton Avenue, Newport, RI 02840.

[Haworth co-indexing entry note]: "Modern Disease Models of Alcoholism and Other Chemical Dependencies: The New Biopsychosocial Models," Wallace, John. Co-published simultaneously in *Drugs & Society* (The Haworth Press, Inc.) Vol. 8, No. 1, 1993, pp. 69-87; and: *Innovations in Alcoholism Treatment: State of the Art Reviews and Their Implications for Clinical Practice* (ed: Gerard J. Connors) The Haworth Press, Inc., 1993, pp. 69-87. Multiple copies of this article/chapter may be purchased from The Haworth Document Delivery Center [1-800-3-HAWORTH; 9:00 a.m. - 5:00 p.m. (EST)].

*69*

many who were afflicted to seek treatment, encouraged the development of adequate funding for research, prevention and treatment services, and secured a place in the American health care system for all chemical dependencies.

At the personal level, the definition of alcoholism as a disease allowed many victims to cope with otherwise overwhelming guilt, remorse, fear, bewilderment, and hopelessness. The concept provided a way for hundreds of thousands of alcoholics to make sense of their experience, to regain a measure of dignity and self-respect, and to begin to take control of and to rebuild their shattered lives. Family members of alcoholics and other chemically dependent people shared in these important psychological benefits. Construing alcoholism as a disease gave many family members the means through which they could stop the self-defeating patterns of self-blaming that go with taking excessive responsibility for the behavior of the other person in the relationship. Moreover, families could be shown a way out of the emotional chaos and intensity that typically accompany life in and around active alcoholism.

The traditional disease concept of alcoholism influenced the ideas of Al-Anon, an organization for the adult significant others of alcoholics. The concept encouraged family members to release the alcoholic with love, take personal responsibility for their own lives, refuse to enable alcoholic behaviors, and to pursue their own individual psychological/spiritual development. These ideas and actions enabled Al-Anon members to deal with their resentments, rage, love-hate conflicts, shattered expectations, and bitterness over the alcoholic behaviors of their partners. Because of the traditional disease concept of alcoholism, many members of Al-Anon became able to forgive the wrongs done them, a necessary first step in their own psychospiritual growth and development and in their own self-healing processes.

In essence, then, the traditional disease concept of alcoholism and other chemical dependencies has provided multifarious individual and societal benefits. More so than any other concept drawn from the medical-biological or sociobehavioral sciences, the traditional disease concept gave rise to nearly a century of progress against alcoholism and served as the basis for the alleviation of suffering for millions of persons who were either directly or indirectly affected by the problem.

## THE DISEASE CONCEPT IN HISTORICAL PERSPECTIVE

The notion that alcoholics should be construed as ill and distinctly different from other drinkers is not a new one. Moreover, this view of alcoholism as a disease did not originate with Alcoholics Anonymous as some critics of that organization have mistakenly claimed. Seneca in ancient Rome drew a distinction between a drunken person and a person who appeared to have no control over repeated drunkenness. Chaucer in 14th Century England came to the same conclusion as Seneca. Neither Seneca nor Chaucer would have accepted the current hypothesis that alcoholism is simply a point on a continuum of alcohol consumption. Both men would have seen alcoholism as a difference in kind and not simply in quantity of consumption.

In 1790, Dr. Benjamin Rush in America wrote about habitual drunkenness as an involuntary condition, a disease caused by "spiritous liquors." "Alcoholism" and "alcohol addiction" were listed in the first American Standard Classified Nomenclature of Disease in 1933 and in every subsequent edition of this widely accepted compilation of diseases. In effect, the traditional disease concept of alcoholism has its roots in ideas present in antiquity as well as in more recent times.

Perhaps one of the more influential variants of the traditional disease concept of alcoholism was contributed by Dr. William Silkworth, the personal physician of Bill Wilson, the founder of Alcoholics Anonymous. Silkworth contributed a chapter to the so-called "Big Book" of AA (Alcoholics Anonymous, 1935) entitled "The Doctor's Opinion." In this chapter, Silkworth, who was not himself an alcoholic, expressed his beliefs about alcoholism thusly: "We believe, and so suggested a few years ago, that the action of alcohol on these chronic alcoholics is a manifestation of an allergy: that the phenomenon of craving is limited to this class and never occurs in the average temperate drinker. These allergic types can never safely use alcohol in any form at all, and once having formed the habit and found they cannot break it, once having lost their self-confidence, their reliance upon things human, their problems pile up on them and become astonishingly difficult to solve" (p. xxvi).

While Silkworth's views on alcoholism and allergy have never been demonstrated to be correct, he had none-the-less made an important contribution. Silkworth had stumbled upon the need for a synthesis of biology and psychology. For Silkworth alcoholism required the joint presence of physical allergy to and mental obsession with alcohol. In a sense, he was the first psychobiologist of alcoholism.

Important further contributions to the traditional disease concept of alcoholism were made by Jellinek (1960) in his now classic work, *Disease Concept of Alcoholism*. Among other things, Jellinek called attention to the heterogeneity of alcoholism and alcohol problems. He attempted to describe this heterogeneity in terms of phases of development of the disease as well as by an hypothesized typology of alcoholic types.

In some sense, it is probably not entirely appropriate to speak of a single traditional disease concept since it is possible to discern a variety of meanings that have been associated with the term. Perhaps the simplest and least arguable meaning concerns the medical consequences of alcoholism. Alcoholism is considered to be a disease by some persons because it is often associated with various diseases, e.g., cirrhosis of the liver, hypertension, pancreatitis, and so forth.

A more sophisticated meaning is simply that alcohol or other drug use produces important biological changes and it is these bodily changes that are linked to further drinking or drug use. Alcohol and other drugs may have profound effects on various brain structures and processes and these effects may mediate further drinking and drug use. Buck and Harris (1991), for example, have recently discussed tolerance and dependence in terms of neuroadaptive responses to chronic ethanol exposure. Ethanol-induced cellular adaptations were considered with regard to GABA receptor-operated chloride channels, voltage sensitive calcium channels, NMDA receptor-operated channels, $G_5$-coupled receptors, and neuronal membranes. The impact of heavy drinking and drug use on various brain neurotransmitter systems and the relationship of such impact to continued heavy use is a further illustration of this meaning of the disease concept.

Still a third meaning that has been associated with the traditional disease concept is that alcoholics and chemically dependent people are biologically different from non-alcoholics and this biological difference preceded the onset of drinking and subsequent dependence. A considerable body of research on genetic influence suggests that this view is at least partially correct. However, as will be pointed out shortly, a pure genetic model that ignores psychological and sociocultural factors is not sufficient for fully explaining the etiology of alcoholism and drug dependence. A more complex model will be described shortly.

## EMERGING CRITICISM

Despite its pragmatic achievements, the traditional disease concept has not been without its detractors, particularly among psychologists and other social-behavioral scientists. For a time, it appeared almost fashionable for psychologists to attack not only various disease models but any and all possible biological factors as well. Marlatt (1983), for example, in a polemic that appeared in the *American Psychologist*, attacked the traditional disease concept with sarcasm:

To some observers, the diagnosis of alcoholism carries the moral stigma of a new scarlet letter. Such critics argue that the contemporary disease model of alcoholism is little more than the old "moral model" (drinking as a sinful behavior) dressed up in sheep's clothing (or at least in a white coat). Despite the fact that the basic tenets of the disease model have yet to be verified scientifically (e.g., the physiological basis of the disease and its primary symptom, loss of control), and even though there is a lack of empirical support for the effectiveness of any particular form of alcoholism treatment (including inpatient programs geared toward abstinence), advocates of the disease model continue to insist that alcoholism is a unitary disorder, a progressive disease that can only be temporarily arrested by total abstention. From this viewpoint, alcohol for the abstinent alcoholic symbolizes the forbidden fruit (a fermented apple?), and a lapse from abstinence is tantamount to a fall from grace in the eyes of God. Clearly, one bite of the forbidden fruit is sufficient to be expelled from paradise. Anyone who suggests controlled drinking is branded as an agent of the devil, tempting the naive alcoholic back into the sin of drinking. If drinking is a sin, the only solution is salvation, a surrendering of personal control to a higher power. (Marlatt, 1983, p. 1107)

Marlatt in this instance revealed the lack of appreciation among psychologists and other social scientists for the extensive body of biological research in alcoholism and other chemical dependencies that has been generated. Moreover, he did not address the lack of rigorous empirical support for the notion that alcoholics and other chemically dependent people in significant numbers can consistently control the level of intoxication in their brains. Even while Marlatt was protesting that biological factors had not been demonstrated, numerous studies in both animal and human genetics had already pointed directly to important genetic biological risk factors or predispositions in the etiology of alcoholism. While such predispositions alone clearly cannot predict the actual development of alcoholism or drug dependence since psychological and sociocultural factors also play important roles, ignoring or denying genetic influences results in an incomplete and inadequate model of these problems.

Marlatt's views on controlled drinking were also incomplete. Recovered alcoholics in Alcoholics Anonymous and clinicians who treat alcoholics do not reject the possibility of controlled intoxication as a recovery or treatment goal for alcoholics because drinking is sinful. They reject controlled intoxication for three reasons: (1) hundreds of thousands of clinical and community observations fail to substantiate the belief that significant numbers of alcohol dependent people are able to engage in long-term, stable, successful controlled intoxication; (2) despite extravagant claims stemming from controlled intoxication research by some psychologists (e.g., Peele, 1988; 1990), rigorous appraisals of this body of research do not support the feasibility of sustained, stable controlled intoxication for alcoholics (e.g., Wallace, 1989a; 1990a); and (3) continued drinking by alcoholics is associated with grave risks for injury, illness, psychological and social negative consequences, and sharply increased mortality. It is also important for some psychologists and other social scientists to realize that Alcoholics Anonymous is not a religious organization. Alcoholics Anonymous refuses to affiliate with any organized religion, has no recognized religious leader, promulgates no religious dogma, and requires its members to believe nothing. The AA program is a broad psychological-spiritual program in which personal and psychospiritual growth are suggested as the means through which persons may achieve freedom from alcohol dependence, restore a lost sense of self, bond to a positive supportive community, develop personal responsibility, gain a positive self-image, and come to view the world with hope, love, and trust rather than pessimism, cynicism, and despair.

Criticism of AA and the traditional disease concept has also characterized the writings of Peele (e.g., 1989a) who regularly inveighs against the traditional disease concept, treatment, abstinence as a proper goal of recovery, and Alcoholics Anonymous. Peele's criticisms, however, seem to be based largely upon strawman arguments and questionable generalizations. His use of strawman argument and extreme statement is apparent in this brief sample of his writings about Alcoholics Anonymous:

> AA preaches a doctrine of total redemption, teetotaling forever. And many a former alcoholic believes that a single drink will send him on the short, slippery slope to alcoholic hell. It's true that for some alcoholics who have been uncontrolled drinkers for many years and whose health has deteriorated, the option of moderation is no longer workable. However, the resolution never to have a drink again is not always a cure-all. The vast majority of alcoholics who try to abstain eventually return to the bottle or to another addiction. (1985, p. 39)

Peele's views on Alcoholics Anonymous are very wide of mark. AA does not "preach a doctrine of total redemption." My own observations of Alcoholics Anonymous number in the thousands. In these many empirical observations made over a quarter of a century in many different locations, I have never heard a single member of AA "preach a doctrine of redemption" (salvation from sin through the atonement of Christ). Moreover, I have never heard a member of Alcoholics Anonymous publicly pledge to "teetotal forever." In actuality, one of the more brilliant tactics of the early members of AA was the simple technique of "time binding." A new member of AA is never encouraged to give up drinking forever but for 24 hours at a time. As members remind each other often, AA is a "day-at-a-time" program, not only with regard to staying sober but for dealing with all of life's problems. Finally, Peele's generalization that the "vast majority of alcoholics who try to abstain eventually return to the bottle or to another addiction" ignores the heterogeneity of alcoholism and the many variables that enter into the course of alcoholism and recovery from it. While Peele's statement may be true of some population of alcoholics, it is certainly not true for all alcoholic populations.

## THE NEED FOR REVISION:
## THE NEW BIOPSYCHOSOCIAL MODELS

Aside from the emotionalism, polemics, ideology, and strawman arguments that have characterized the writings of some critics of the traditional disease concept, it is evident that the concept must necessarily undergo continuous revision in light of several decades of research and clinical observation. Fortunately, more moderate voices can also be heard in the call for necessary revision.

Perhaps the most significant development in recent years has been the growing recognition that critics need not attempt to refute all possible biological factors and the recovery goal of abstention in order to achieve comprehensive and even more pragmatic models of alcoholism and other chemical dependencies. Integrative models that build upon the strengths of the past and recognize the validity of various levels of analysis and disciplinary efforts are now available. These new integrative disease models are biopsychosocial models. They are based on the fact that it is now abundantly clear that biological, behavioral, cognitive, psychosocial, and sociocultural events all enter into the nature of alcoholism and addictive diseases of all types. Biopsychosocial models are a refreshing alternative to the unfortunate "nothing butism" that has characterized the debate over theoretical models of alcoholism and encouraged nonproductive pseudo-controversies that have generated more heat than light. "Nothing butism" refers to the tendency for certain persons to argue that alcoholism is nothing but learned behavior, *or* nothing but a genetic disorder, *or* nothing but a product of expectations and beliefs, *or* nothing but a disease, *or* nothing but a cultural phenomenon. All such statements are rightfully regarded as narrow and partial and incapable of explaining what is clearly a multidimensional phenomenon. Moreover, it has become increasingly clear that it is fruitless to continue to cast the issues in terms of various dichotomies, e.g., "Is alcoholism learned or inherited?" "Is alcoholism biological or psychological?" "Is alcoholism a product of expectancies or is it the pharmacology of the drug?" and so on and so forth.

In recognition of the need for more comprehensive multidimensional models, attention is now turning to biopsychosocial models. Early work on biopsychosocial models was contributed by Ewing (1983), Tarter (1983) and Wallace (1983a; 1984; 1985; 1989b; 1990b), all of whom called for such models as the next logical step in the development of more sophisticated and accurate models of alcoholism and other chemical dependencies.

The advantages of biopsychosocial models over the traditional disease concept are numerous. First, and perhaps most important, biopsychosocial models are inclusive rather than exclusive. Such models encourage free exploration within, between, and among important scientific/clinical disciplines. From biopsychosocial perspectives, biological, psychological, and sociocultural phenomena are all regarded as important domains of study for scientists and clinicians. Widespread adoption of biopsychosocial models would do much to reduce the ideological clashes that have characterized the field of alcoholism, encouraging respect rather than distrust and disdain across disciplines and recovery approaches.

Second, biopsychosocial models are clearly necessary as it has become increasingly evident that a naive disease concept is untenable in light of several decades of research. In short, biopsychosocial models fit reality far better than any single dimensional model drawn from biological, psychological, or sociocultural domains alone.

Third, biopsychosocial models will encourage needed interdisciplinary collaborative efforts. Obviously, psychologists and neurobiologists have much to contribute to each other as do anthropologists and geneticists. Alcoholism and chemical dependencies in general are simply too complex to be comprehended merely as a behavioral problem, or a matter of expectancies, or cultural surrounds, or brain chemistry. Progress in the next decade will come from scientists and clinicians from different disciplines working on integrative models that utilize multiple theoretical languages and levels of analysis.

## UTILIZING BIOPSYCHOSOCIAL MODELS IN CHEMICAL DEPENDENCE TREATMENT

Treatment programs that operate out of single dimensional models fail to inform and treat patients from a comprehensive perspective. When the focus is upon behavior only, important information concerning such things as the neurochemical basis for craving for a drug like cocaine can go unappreciated. Cocaine dependent patients, for example, need to understand that the drug acts as a dopamine reuptake blocker and that this is the basis for the initial euphoria associated with the drug in the early period of use. As use deepens and extends over time, however, dopamine depletion at synaptic levels begins to occur, proliferation of dopamine receptors takes place, supersensitivity of the dopamine system appears, neurotransmitters other than dopamine are similarly affected, and the initial euphoria is either replaced or followed quickly by anhedonia (e.g., Wallace, 1988). These brain events are also associated with increased craving for the drug, briefer highs, depression, self-disregard, agitation, irresponsibility, and paranoid thinking. In short, the cocaine dependent patient needs to come to understand the almost certain readdiction to the drug that will occur as a function of changes in brain chemistry if use is again attempted. The patient also needs to understand the brain chemistry involved in cocaine use and dependence in order to grasp the limited usefulness of concepts such as will power, character, and controlled cocaine use in the face of cocaine dependence.

But while the patient must come to understand the chemistry of addiction, he or she must also come to appreciate the learning and conditioning involved in addiction. Behavioral analysis suggests quite strongly that stimuli present when cocaine is used can acquire the strength to elicit craving for the drug. Hence, things like mirrors, straws, baking soda, razor blades, vials of crack, and so forth operate as conditioned stimuli for use.

Both the neurochemistry of addiction and the conditioning of addiction have direct treatment implications other than education of patients. Psychopharmacological research may lead to important drug or nutritional interventions aimed at the dopamine and other neurotransmitter systems. On the other hand, learning theory has given rise to important new research on "cue exposure" and other behavioral approaches to reducing the power of conditioned stimuli to elicit craving and drug use. The point is that neither the biological or psychological explanations is the correct one. Rather, both sets of explanations can lead to important and potentially useful interventions and can provide patients with useful "cognitive maps" of the nature of the problem with which they must deal. This analysis could also be extended to include understandings about the patient's natural social environment outside of the treatment setting. Friendship, lover, and marital choices and relationships are important factors that patients must consider. Trying to stay clean and sober while immersed in relationships with heavy drinking and drug using persons is not likely to work. Or, to take a more dramatic example, one does not encourage addicts and alcoholics to hang out in crack houses and bars. Obviously, the social environment is as critical as the brain's neurotransmitter systems in determining use, dependence, and relapse.

Biopsychosocial models require clinicians to present information to patients in a manner that encourages deeper appreciation of the issues involved. It is, for example, most inappropriate for clinicians to inform their patients that alcoholism *per se* is an inherited condition. It is necessary for clinicians to explain that an "alcogene" that inevitably drives persons into alcoholism has not yet been identified. Rather, patients should be taught the following about alcoholism as a genetically *influenced* disease:

1. alcoholism is polygenic, i.e., numerous genes are involved in its development;
2. multiple biologic risk factors may predispose persons to the illness;
3. the presence of biologic risk factors for alcoholism does not inevitably drive a person into alcoholism since culture, society, and other environmental factors may override the genetic push;
4. not all persons with alcohol or drug problems show a family history for the illness and this suggests that pathways into the problem other than a genetic/biological one may exist;
5. the existence of biological predispositions for alcoholism and drug addiction should not render us hopeless in the face of the illness since environmental factors can without question importantly influence the course and expression of the disease.

Patients should also be taught that while biological risk factors for alcoholism (and other drug dependencies) do exist and can be transmitted genetically, the nature of these risk factors are still far from clear. Research, however, has pointed to important new hypotheses. In alcoholism, for example, a considerable body of animal and human evidence suggests a problem in the serotonin neurotransmitter receptor system for at least some alcoholics. Genetic strains of alcohol preferring rats, for example, show consistent defects in serotonin levels in particular brain structures (Li et al., 1987). Moreover, experimental manipulations of serotonin levels in both animals and humans have revealed an inverse relationship between drinking of alcohol and serotonin levels (e.g., Naranjo et al., 1984). Even with such impressive and consistent findings, however, care must be exercised in explaining the etiology of alcoholism to patients in terms of the serotonin hypothesis. It is possible, for example, that the serotonin deficiency effect is not specific to alcoholism but may involve consummatory behavior in general. Moreover, deficits in hypothalamic serotonin may impact upon drinking of any fluids (not only alcohol) through thirst regulation via the renin-angiotensin system. To complicate matters further, it has been demonstrated recently that while fluid intake in general is inversely related to plasma renin activity levels, so is alcohol intake (Kalant & Leenen, 1989).

Neurotransmitters other than serotonin have been implicated in alcoholism. Borg and colleagues in Sweden, for example, have studied the role of noradrenaline and have reported that relapse back into active alcoholism for some alcoholics was preceded by a fall in noradrenaline in Swedish alcoholics. These and other data have led Wallace (1989b) to speculate that an arousal/activation deviation may exist and may serve as the basis for two types of alcoholics, i.e., the hyperaroused alcoholic and the hypoaroused. According to Wallace's hypothesis, hyperaroused alcoholics suffer from excessive arousal/activation and show characteristic signs of various anxiety diseases and disorders as well as obsessive compulsive illness. Drinking and drug taking in these patients is thought to be aimed at reducing excessive levels of arousal. Such patients are often also drawn to sedative drugs like the benzodiazepines and barbiturates.

On the other hand, hypoaroused alcoholics may represent a distinctly different population who seek out the stimulating properties of impromptu drinking situations, uninhibited drunken comportment, and the "action" available in bars and on the streets. These alcoholics are likely to suffer from anhedonia rather than from excessive fear, worry, anxiety, or obsessive thoughts. They tend toward simultaneous heavy use of central nervous system stimulants such as cocaine, amphetamines and crack.

In effect, Wallace suggests that treatment requirements may vary significantly for these two hypothesized types of patients. In the one case, the central goal of treatment is to teach the patient strategies and behaviors for reducing excessive arousal/activation levels. Meditation, relaxation training, autohypnosis, biofeedback, heavy immersion in non-threatening highly supportive 12-step recovery programs, and so forth may prove optimal. Possible pharmacologic treatments for very severe cases might involve low dose desipramine treatment for panic disorder, non-benzodiazepine anxiolytics such as buspirone hydrochloride, clomipramine for obsessive compulsive disorder, and cardiac drugs like the nonaddictive calcium channel blocker verapamil or the beta blocker inderal may find important further uses in alcoholism treatment.

For hypoaroused patients, however, different treatment strategies may prove necessary. Such patients may require considerable therapeutic effort directed at dealing with painful states of anhedonia, boredom, restlessness, and stimulation-seeking in recovery. Such patients may need to learn how to seek out and engage in non-drug situations and activities that arouse and excite rather than those situations that calm and relax. Exercise, dancing, sporting events, outdoor adventures, risk-taking, novel situations, contact games and sports, aviation, parachuting, and so forth may be important supplements to 12-step program involvement and other recovery activities for patients who tend toward hypoaroused states when free of alcohol and drugs.

Aside from possible neurotransmitter system differences between alcoholics and non-alcoholics, biologic research has also examined enzymatic differences (Tabakoff et al., 1988), aldehyde-neurotransmitter condensation products (Myers, 1985), brain electrical activity (Begleiter & Porjesz, 1988), and neuronal membranes and ion channels (Goldstein, 1983). Tarter et al. (1990) have developed intriguing ideas concerning inherited deviations in temperament traits that may be linked to the etiology of alcoholism. Behavioral activity regulation appears to be the inherited temperament trait of greatest importance in alcoholism.

With regard to treatment, all of this recent information concerning neurotransmitters, enzymes, aldehyde-neurotransmitter condensation products, brain electrical activity, and temperament traits can be shared with patients to help them to understand the possible biological factors in their illnesses, and also why many refer to alcoholism and drug dependencies as diseases.

## PSYCHOLOGICAL FACTORS
## AND BIOPSYCHOSOCIAL MODELS

Programs that have incorporated the traditional disease model have not, as a rule, neglected psychological factors. Alcoholics Anonymous, for example, is very much a program of behavior, cognitive and personality change. Direct observations of AA members and meeting behaviors would quickly verify the fact that AA is indeed a psychological as well as a spiritual program of recovery. Wallace (1983b) has pointed out the many psychological concerns of AA members, e.g., resentments toward others, self-pity, fear, anger, envy, sexual needs, social recognition and ego needs, self-concept and self-esteem, impulse control, security needs, approval needs, and so forth. Such things as these are frequently discussed at meetings.

Moreover, as Wallace (1983b) has indicated, AA incorporates many sound principles of behavior, cognitive, and personality change that are not at all incompatible with modern psychological therapies. Reinforcement theory, social learning theory, cognitive behavioral change theory, and reference group theory are clearly evident in the practices of AA groups and, AA, in fact, appears to have anticipated these developments by formal, academic psychologists by many years. In short, AA has been much kinder to psychological thought than many of its critics have realized. Despite many AA members' beliefs in some variant of the traditional disease model, it is abundantly clear that their programs of recovery are heavily saturated with sound psychological theories and practices. In light of these observations, it is difficult to understand why the critics of AA, for the most part, have been academic psychologists.

Biopsychosocial models can be expected to permit the further development of psychological theory and practices in the chemical dependence field. Valuable technologies drawn from behavioral and cognitive research may very well enhance current treatment models.

Finally, with regard to psychological issues, biopsychosocial models can readily accommodate recent interest in dually diagnosed patients. As alcoholic patients often were poorly served in mental health clinics and hospitals, dual diagnosis patients often have been poorly served in alcoholism specialty units. Biopsychosocial models would provide the means for mental health and alcoholism treatment workers to strip away the ideological blinders that have often prevented both from seeing the patient as he or she actually is.

## SOCIOCULTURAL SURROUNDS

Perhaps the greatest contribution that biopsychosocial models can make at this time is to raise awareness as to the importance of social and cultural factors in the origins and maintenance of alcoholism and other drug dependence. Among the republics of the Soviet Union, for example, alcohol problems vary from a low of 1% in some republics to a high of roughly 20% in others. Surely a substantial portion of this variability can be attributed to sociocultural differences.

With regard to alcoholism treatment, considerably more attention must be paid to the environments to which patients are returned after residential treatment. And for patients in outpatient treatment, attention must be drawn to the extra-treatment factors that exert so much influence on behavior. There is evidence that the environments to which patients return after residential treatment account for as much of the variability in treatment outcome as do the characteristics they bring to treatment in combination with treatment itself (Billings & Moos, 1983).

A limitation of the traditional disease model has been its virtual neglect of sociocultural factors. But as I have argued, it is not necessary to throw the biological baby out with the bath of cultural relativity. Both biology and culture can co-exist and, in fact, complement each other. Only those who suffer from rather advanced hardening of the categories will insist on keeping them separate.

Genetic predispositions, for example, do not unfold in a cultural vacuum. It is entirely possible to inherit multiple predispositions to alcoholism but escape the disease altogether if one happens to be born and raised in a society or culture with strict prohibitions against alcohol consumption. On the other hand, a person with exactly the same set of predispositions would be a prime candidate for full blown alcoholism in a society and culture in which heavy drinking is not only tolerated but encouraged. Biologic factors may predispose but society and culture may control the very important element of degree of *exposure* to the chemicals. Family systems, community characteristics, cultural diversity, and societal customs and mores concerning drinking and drug use are all legitimate subjects of inquiry in various biopsychosocial models. Such things were either ignored completely or considered only partially in the traditional disease concept.

# THE NEW DISEASE MODELS:
# IS THERE REALLY AN ARGUMENT?

The acceptance of multidimensional, biopsychosocial disease models of alcoholism and chemical dependence that incorporate events from all levels of analysis makes much of the debate over *the* correct unidimensional model rather meaningless. Psychologists will simply have to come to terms with the reality of biological factors of many kinds in alcoholism and chemical dependence. On the other hand, traditional disease concept theorists will have to make more room in their conceptual maps for psychological theories and techniques. Both groups will need to learn greater openness to the societal and cultural levels of analysis where much work remains to be done.

In short, it is time for the various unidimensional camps to realize that the ideological skirmishes that have characterized the chemical dependence field are largely pointless and nonproductive. The real questions are now substantive. What are the biological risk factors that make up genetic predisposition? How do psychological factors enter into the maintenance of alcoholism and other drug dependence? How can study of societal variables and cultural phenomena lead us to effective prevention strategies? And most important, how can these many factors at different levels of analysis be combined into multidimensional integrated models with substantial explanatory power?

It is not that the notion of alcoholism as a disease is no longer useful and must be abandoned. The notion must be enlarged, enriched, and expanded. The interplay between and among biology, psychology, and society and culture is now recognized for many diseases other than alcoholism and chemical dependence. Psychological factors, for example, may impact significantly on the immune system and hence, upon a large number of diseases including cancer. Societal and cultural factors in food selection and dietary practices may have important implications for coronary artery disease. Biological factors may underlie psychological problems like panic disorder, mood disturbances, and anorexia. In effect, biopsychosocial models are proving useful in describing the etiology and maintenance of many diseases.

This realization of the importance of interacting biological, psychological and sociocultural dimensions is one of the more exciting developments in modern medicine. Surely this realization will be extended to alcoholism and chemical dependence as well.

## REFERENCES

Alcoholics Anonymous. (1976). New York: Alcoholics Anonymous World Services.

Begleiter, H., & Porjesz, B. (1988). Potential biological markers in individuals at high risk for developing alcoholism. *Alcoholism: Clinical and Experimental Research, 12*, 488-493.

Billings, A., & Moos, R. (1983). Psychosocial processes of recovery among alcoholics and their families: Implications for clinicians and program evaluators. *Addictive Behaviors, 8*, 205-218.

Borg, S., Kvande, H., & Sedvall, G. (1981). Central norepinephrine metabolism during alcohol intoxication in addicts and healthy volunteers. *Science, 213*, 1136-1137.

Buck, K.J., & Harris, R.A. (June, 1991). Neuroadaptive responses to chronic ethanol. *Alcoholism: Clinical and Experimental Research, 15*, 460-471.

Ewing, J.A. (1983). Alcoholism–Another biopsychosocial disease. *Psychosomatics, 21*, 371-372.

Goldstein, D.B. (1983). *Pharmacology of alcohol.* New York: Oxford University Press.

Jellinek, E.M. (1960). *Disease concept of alcoholism.* New Haven, CT: United Printing Service.

Kalant, H., & Leenen, F. (1989). Alcohol intake is inversely related to plasma renin activity in the genetically selected alcohol-preferring and nonpreferring lines of rats. *Pharmacology Biochemistry & Behavior, 32*, 1061-1063.

Li, T.K., Lumeng, L., McBride, W.J. et al. (1987). Rodent lines selected for factors affecting alcohol consumption. *Alcohol and Alcoholism,* Supplement Vol. 1, 91-96.

Marlatt, G.A. (1983). The controlled drinking controversy: A commentary. *American Psychologist, 38*, 1098-1110.

Myers, R.D. (1985). Multiple metabolite theory, alcohol drinking, and the alcogene. In M.A. Collins (Ed.), *Aldehyde adducts in alcoholism* (pp. 201-220). New York: Alan R. Liss.

Naranjo, C.A., Sellers, C.M., Roach, C.A. et al. (1984). Zimelidine-induced variations in alcohol intake by nondepressed heavy drinkers. *Clinical Pharmacological Therapeutics, 35*, 374-381.

Peele, S. (1988). Can alcoholism and other addiction problems be treated away or is the current treatment binge doing more harm than good? *Journal of Psychoactive Drugs, 20*, 375-383.

Peele, S. (1989). *Diseasing of America–Addiction treatment out of control.* Lexington, MA: Lexington Books.

Peele, S. (1990). Why and by whom the American alcoholism treatment industry is under siege. *Journal of Psychoactive Drugs, 22,* 1-13.

Tabakoff, B., Hoffman, P.L., Lee, J.M. et al. (1988). Differences in platelet enzyme activity between alcoholics and nonalcoholics. *New England Journal of Medicine, 318,* 134-139.

Tarter, R.E. (1983). The causes of alcoholism: A biopsychosocial analysis. In E. Gottheil, K. Druley, T. Skolada, & H. Waxman (Eds.), *Etiological aspects of alcohol and drug abuse.* Springfield, IL: Charles C. Thomas.

Tarter, R.E., Laird, S.B., Mostefa, K., Burkstein, O., & Kaminer, Y. (1990). Drug abuse severity in adolescents is associated with magnitude of deviation in temperament traits. *British Journal of Addiction, 85,* 1501-1504.

Wallace, J. (1983a). Alcoholism: Is a shift in paradigm necessary? *Journal of Psychiatric Treatment and Evaluation, 5,* 479-485.

Wallace, J. (1983b). Ideology, belief, and behavior: Alcoholics Anonymous as a social movement. In E. Gottheil, K. Druley, T. Skolada, & H. Waxman (Eds.), *Etiological aspects of alcohol and drug abuse.* Springfield, IL: Charles C. Thomas.

Wallace, J. (1984). Frontiers of biopsychosocial research: Filling in the biological dimension. *Westchester Alcoholism Reporter, 6,* 1-3.

Wallace, J. (1985). Predicting the onset of compulsive drinking in alcoholics: A biopsychosocial model. *Alcohol, 2,* 589-595.

Wallace, J. (1988). The relevance to clinical care of recent research in neurobiology. *Journal of Substance Abuse Treatment, 5,* 207-217.

Wallace, J. (1989a). Can Stanton Peele's opinions be taken seriously? A reply to Peele. *Journal of Psychoactive Drugs, 21,* 259-271.

Wallace, J. (1989b). A biopsychosocial model of alcoholism. *Social Casework, 70,* 325-332.

Wallace, J. (1990a). Controlled drinking, treatment effectiveness, and the disease model of addiction: A commentary on the ideological wishes of Stanton Peele. *Journal of Psychoactive Drugs, 22,* 261-284.

Wallace, J. (1990b). The new disease model of alcoholism. *The Western Journal of Medicine, 152,* 502-505.

# Sociocultural Aspects
# of Alcohol Use and Abuse:
# Ethnicity and Gender

## R. Lorraine Collins

**SUMMARY.** This review focuses on ethnicity and gender as key components of a sociocultural perspective on alcohol use and abuse. Conceptual issues in the use of ethnic categorization, particularly as they relate to the failure to examine differences within groups, are highlighted. Research on the prevalence of use, primary prevention, and treatment is reviewed and recommendations for future research are outlined. It is concluded that more careful attention to the impact of sociocultural factors, rather than the reliance on ethnic and gender based comparisons, will add to the knowledge gained from research on alcohol use and abuse.

Sociocultural factors are important in alcohol research as there is much variation in patterns of use and reactions to alcohol. Some of these variations are related to aspects of culture and social organization. There are a number of variables that can be conceptualized as representing sociocultural factors in alcohol use. In the present article, I will focus on ethnicity (the four major non-European ethnic groups that reside in the U.S.: African-Americans, American-Indians, Asian-Americans, and Latinos) as well as gender (women)

---

R. Lorraine Collins is affiliated with the Research Institute on Addictions, 1021 Main Street, Buffalo, NY 14203.

[Haworth co-indexing entry note]: "Sociocultural Aspects of Alcohol Use and Abuse: Ethnicity and Gender," Collins, R. Lorraine. Co-published simultaneously in *Drugs & Society* (The Haworth Press, Inc.) Vol. 8, No. 1, 1993, pp. 89-116; and: *Innovations in Alcoholism Treatment: State of the Art Reviews and Their Implications for Clinical Practice* (ed: Gerard J. Connors) The Haworth Press, Inc., 1993, pp. 89-116. Multiple copies of this article/chapter may be purchased from The Haworth Document Delivery Center [1-800-3-HAWORTH; 9:00 a.m. - 5:00 p.m. (EST)].

as key components of a sociocultural perspective on alcohol use. Research on prevalence, primary prevention, and treatment of alcohol use/abuse among ethnic populations and women will be used to illustrate our current state of knowledge, and to discuss potential areas for future research.

Consideration of ethnicity and gender as sociocultural factors has a long history in alcohol research. For example, MacAndrew and Edgerton's (1969) seminal work on drunken behavior among different peoples indicated that sociocultural factors accounted for much of the variation in patterns of alcohol use as well as in the behaviors exhibited while "under the influence" of alcohol. This work has had a major influence on research concerning cognitive factors in alcohol use (e.g., Critchlow, 1986; Marlatt & Rohsenow, 1980) and has contributed to the development of the social-learning perspective on alcohol use/abuse (e.g., Wilson, 1988). In the current research climate, attention to ethnicity as a sociocultural factor has often been reduced to comparative studies in which European-Americans (as the numerical and cultural majority) have served as the standard to which other (numerically smaller) non-European ethnic groups have been compared. In addition, descriptive studies of ethnic and gender-related differences in alcohol use have added little to theory development and/or the conceptual complexity of notions concerning the prevalence of alcohol use, effective primary prevention, and the treatment of alcohol abuse.

## ETHNICITY AS A SOCIOCULTURAL FACTOR IN ALCOHOL RESEARCH

The complexity of the task of conducting research on a variety of ethnic groups begins with conceptualization of the term ethnicity. In the U.S., researchers and policy makers have sought to simplify the designation of ethnicity, but in so doing have reduced its meaningfulness. Heath (1990-91) described five garbled versions of ethnicity including ethnicity as race (garbling based on biology) and ethnicity as national heritage (garbling based on politics), each of which was "imprecise and unreliable" (p. 607).

Race is a particularly compelling designation in the U.S. Possibly as a reflection of the preoccupation with race within the broader society, racial categories often are used in alcohol research, where it is common to see references to "White" and "Black" subjects, as if these designations had scientific meaning or validity. Race is not an objective, biological category, but rather a social category (Cheung, 1989; Fisher, 1987; Heath, 1990-91). Physical characteristics that stereotypically determine racial identity (skin color, eye shape, texture of hair) each vary along a continuum and can be combined in an almost infinite number of configurations. In fact, racial categories common in the U.S. are not homogeneous, but rather encompass a range of variation in physical characteristics, education, social status, and cultural background. This variation within racial categories as well as the fact that variables other than race (e.g., gender, socioeconomic status) may be more important in determining drinking behavior has led Heath (1990-91) to declare "the racial model of ethnicity in alcohol studies is bankrupt" (p. 617).

Ethnicity has been selected as a more comprehensive and seemingly more representative designation since it involves notions of a shared culture or identity. However, in many cases ethnic labels have been used interchangeably with racial designations, resulting in a similar set of superficial and simplistic categories. The resulting "ethnic glosses" (Trimble, 1990-91) are not informative because they too are not homogeneous. For most groups, ethnic glosses mask important differences in national origins, cultural traditions, and other variables. For example, Latinos are composed of populations from Cuba, Puerto Rico, Mexico, as well as Central and South America. Each of these populations has a different history and set of traditions in their countries of origin as well as within the U.S. As a reflection of these factors, Caetano (1986) found differences in drinking patterns and social position based on the specific definition of Latino/Hispanic ethnicity used in a national survey of alcohol use. Similarly, Asian-Americans are composed of populations from various countries in South East Asia, China, and Japan. Further, some Asian-Americans are new to the U.S. and some have lived in the U.S. for many generations. The designation "American-Indian" includes over 400 tribes recognized by the U.S. Bureau of Indian Affairs. As with racial designations, other sources of heterogeneity within ethnic groups include gender, education, acculturation, age, and socioeconomic status (SES); each of these variables is independently related to alcohol use (Caetano, 1986; Collins, 1992).

To further complicate the picture, ethnic/cultural identity may not exist only as a category or on a continuum, as is typical of the approaches used in alcohol research, but perhaps may be best viewed as orthogonal (Oetting & Beauvais, 1990-91). This orthogonal conceptualization means that persons can identify equally strongly (or weakly) with two cultures, adding even more to the misinformation provided by the use of an ethnic gloss. In their data on American-Indian adolescents, Oetting and Beauvais found that strong identification with American-Indian culture, European-American culture, or both cultures had positive relationships to characteristics such as self-esteem. In fact, the highest self-esteem was found in those adolescents who strongly identified with both cultures. The relationships between cultural identification and substance use were inconsistent and seemed to be related to other factors such as peer influences. However, both the orthogonal conceptualization and these findings suggest that some individuals possess a complex sense of cultural identity that cannot easily be categorized. Thus, the use of ethnic glosses as proxies for cultural identity is not likely to be meaningful.

The use of ethnic glosses typically has been designated a methodological issue that impacts on the replication of studies and/or the external validity of findings (Collins, 1992; Trimble 1990-91). In fact, the use of such glosses must be considered more broadly as a conceptual issue that creates core problems in the conduct and interpretation of research. The limited utility of ethnic categories raises some fundamental issues vis-à-vis alcohol research. First, it raises questions about the conceptual maturity of psychosocial research on alcohol use, since ethnic categories typically provide only a context for describing drinking behavior, but offer little if anything in terms of consistent explanations of drinking. Heath (1990-91), for example, has suggested that ethnicity research has highlighted the role of social learning as a basis for various aspects of drinking. However, few researchers have developed models that explain how sociocultural characteristics may relate to specific drinking patterns within groups.

A related question concerns the continuing emphasis on ethnicity-based research when variables other than ethnicity may better account for the variance in drinking behavior. For example, Oetting and Beauvais (1987b) have reported that peer influences on drug use do not differ for Mexican-American, American-Indian, and European-American adolescents. Given the similarity in the peer socialization process among these three groups, it would seem that variables other than ethnicity might be a more meaningful basis for considering alcohol-related behavior. Although findings of similarities across groups are helping to underscore the limited utility of ethnic categories, this type of research represents limited progress. Many researchers still cling to ethnic labels and fail to include explanatory variables that could account for findings both within and between groups. This being the state-of-the-art, I am left with the dilemma of acknowledging the limitations of ethnic glosses while reviewing research that makes use of such glosses. One can only hope that this state of affairs will change in the future.

One of the sources of heterogeneity both within and between sociocultural groupings is the group's structural position in the broader society. This typically refers to the group's level of social organization, which allows it to compete with other groups for resources and power within the institutions of the larger society (Cheung, 1989). Generally, a group's structural position is related to its socioeconomic position in society, which in turn, is linked to drinking behavior. For example, the results from general population surveys typically indicate differences in drinking based on income. Thus, Midanik and Room (1992) reported that in a representative national sample, the percentage of drinkers increased from a low of 68% among those with a yearly family income under $9,000 to a high of around 79% for those with a yearly family income of $40,000 or more. However, rates of heavier drinking (5+ drinks/day) were much higher in the low income sample (19%) than in the high income sample (6%). Midanik and Room found a similar pattern for education; specifically, a higher proportion of drinkers, but less heavy drinking, among the better educated. These data suggest that drinking varies with social position, with those of lower SES being at higher risk for alcohol-related problems.

In the U.S., historical and social events have combined to create a situation in which large proportions of members of some non-European ethnic groups are of lower socioeconomic status. This has resulted in a tendency for behaviors related to the preponderance of low SES members to be stereotypically generalized to the entire group. It also has meant that alcohol-related social problems that reflect the lack of access to economic resources and social power are attributed to enduring psychological (or even biological) characteristics of the group. More generally, this state of affairs is reflected in a tendency to confound ethnicity/race with social class, such that ethnicity is used to explain behaviors that actually vary based on class (Cheung, 1989; Collins, 1992; Fisher, 1987).

Interestingly, many studies on alcohol use/abuse still fail to include even a rudimentary description or analysis of sociocultural characteristics such as SES, and some researchers seem comfortable ascribing differences to ethnicity rather than considering the impact of the socioeconomic position of the groups being studied. When socioeconomic position is considered, it has been shown to play an explanatory role. Thus, in Wallace and Bachman's (1991) analysis of sociocultural factors in drug use (including alcohol) among a large, multi-ethnic sample of high school seniors, it was found that drug use among American-Indians was linked to socioeconomic status. Wallace and Bachman state "the data suggest that the higher than average level of drug use reported by Native American youth may be linked to their relatively disadvantaged socioeconomic status. Once the background differences were adjusted, the white versus Native American differences in drug use are virtually eliminated among male seniors and reduced or eliminated among female seniors" (p. 343). Rhodes and Jason (1990) have made a similar argument with regard to the socioeconomic disadvantages faced by urban African-American and Hispanic adolescents.

Osborne and Feit's (1992) assessment of the failure to assess and consider the role of sociocultural factors in medical research is applicable to the state-of-the-art in alcohol research. They state "ethnic categorization in medical research projects the misleading implication that race is a more important determinant of disease than class, lifestyle, or socioeconomic status" (p. 276). Which raises the following question: If socioeconomic status and other sociocultural variables are important in determining alcohol use, why are we not seeing more research in which these variables play central roles as possible explanations for alcohol-related outcomes? These and other issues relevant to ethnicity will be considered in my discussion of sociocultural factors in research on prevalence of alcohol use, prevention of alcohol problems, and alcohol treatment.

## GENDER AS A SOCIOCULTURAL FACTOR IN ALCOHOL RESEARCH

Research on the role of gender in alcohol use/abuse also raises many of the issues addressed in our consideration of ethnicity. Even with the more objective biological criteria for designating gender, within group variations in drinking behavior also occur. For example, sex-role orientation of men and women may account for more variation in the drinking behavior of some samples than does biological gender (Chomak & Collins, 1987). Other sources of variation in the drinking behavior of men and women include: (1) marital status (Wilsnack, Wilsnack, & Klassen, 1985), (2) age and life roles (Fillmore, 1987; Midanik & Room, 1992; NIAAA, 1990); (3) employment and income (Midanik & Room, 1992; Wilsnack et al., 1985); and (4) education (Midanik & Room, 1992). In general population surveys, men typically report drinking more than women and have more alcohol-related problems regardless of race, ethnicity, or age (Hilton, 1987; Lex, 1991; Midanik & Room, 1992). However, the differences between the alcohol intake of men and women decline somewhat when adjustment for body weight and body water are made (Chomak & Collins, 1987; Dawson & Archer, 1992). Even so, social sanctions against women's drinking as well as women's generally lower social position have resulted in decreased alcohol consumption.

Women's biological heritage and social roles have created certain unique issues that must be considered in alcohol research (Collins, 1992). These include the role of alcohol in female sexuality and reproduction (e.g., fetal alcohol syndrome), the possible impact of victimization on women's development of alcohol problems (Hurley, 1991; Miller, Downs, Gondoli, & Keil, 1987), and the barriers to women's participation in alcoholism treatment (Beckman & Amaro, 1984; Thom, 1986). Issues unique to women also will be considered in the following discussion of sociocultural factors in research on the prevalence of alcohol use, prevention, and treatment of alcohol problems.

## OVERVIEW OF RESEARCH
## ON THE PREVALENCE OF ALCOHOL ABUSE

Much of the data on the prevalence of alcohol use and abuse is collected in large national epidemiological surveys such as the Monitoring the Future (a yearly survey of substance use among high school students; e.g., Johnson, O'Malley, & Bachman, 1992) and the National Health and Nutrition Examination Survey (NHANES). Some surveys oversample ethnic populations or focus on under-represented groups (Colliver, Grigson, Barbano, Dufour, & Malin, 1989). For example, the Hispanic Health and Nutrition Examination Survey (HHANES) was an offshoot of the NHANES that included representative samples of Cuban-Americans from Dade County Florida, Puerto-Ricans living in the New York City area, and Mexican-Americans living in the southwest (Christian, Zobeck, Malin, & Hitchcock, 1989). Generally, the results of national surveys indicate a decline in the total amount of alcohol being consumed in the U.S., with decreases in hard liquor and relative stability in wine and beer consumption (NIAAA, 1990). Summaries of the drinking patterns of ethnic groups indicate that African-Americans have relatively high rates of abstention. However, high rates of heavy drinking among certain subgroups of African-Americans, particularly middle aged men and women, have contributed to a high incidence of alcohol-related health problems. Asian-Americans generally exhibit low levels of alcohol use and abuse. American-Indians exhibit high rates of alcohol use and abuse and experience more alcohol-related health and social problems. Latino men have a high rate of alcohol use and abuse, but many Latino women abstain from alcohol. These general patterns vary based on psychosocial characteristics such as age and gender (NIAAA, 1990).

In almost every ethnic group, more men drink alcohol than do women (Gilbert & Collins, in press). However, there are variations within and between groups. For example, among African-Americans drinking generally decreases with age, with particularly high levels of abstention (60% or more) for women and men at age 60 or older. At all age levels, women drink less than men and exhibit higher levels of abstention. However, for both African-American women and men, lifetime prevalence of alcohol abuse is highest in middle age. Herd's (1989) comprehensive description of drinking behavior of national samples of African-Americans indicated regional variations in drinking as well as the impact of sociocultural factors such as religiosity.

American-Indians have stereotypically been seen as being at high risk for alcohol abuse (NIAAA, 1990). However, variations in cultural practices and tribal affiliation are related to the prevalence of alcohol abuse. In most tribes, men drink more than women and have more alcohol-related problems (Leland, 1984; May & Smith, 1988). One interesting deviation from this pattern was found among members of the Sioux tribe, where men and women tended to drink similar amounts (Weibel-Orlando, 1989). Although drinking among the Navajo decreased with age, alcohol-related problems were seen in all age groups (May & Smith, 1988). Other variables that may impact on drinking behavior of American-Indians are location (urban Indians may drink more that rural Indians; Weibel-Orlando, 1989) and level of employment (unemployed drink more than employed; Lex, 1987).

Asian-Americans have stereotypically been seen as drinking less than the general population and therefore having fewer alcohol problems. As a reflection of this notion and the related paucity of research on Asian-Americans in alcoholism treatment, Asians are typically not included in reviews of alcohol problems among non-European ethnic groups (e.g., Lex, 1987). While the stereotypes about Asian drinking may be true for some subgroups, the drinking behavior of Asian-Americans is quite varied. Sources of variation include gender, country of origin, and level of acculturation. In most Asian groups, men show much higher rates of drinking than women. Thus, among Filipinos living in Los Angeles, 81% of men were drinkers while only 45% of women drank (Lubben, Chi, & Kitano, 1988). However, there are some consistencies regarding drinking norms that may impact on women and men. Japanese have relatively tolerant drinking norms for men and Japanese-Americans have more egalitarian norms regarding women's drinking. Possibly as a result of these factors, Japanese-American men (29%) and women (12%) exhibited the highest rates of heavy drinking among a sample of Japanese, Chinese, and Koreans living in Los Angeles (Chi, Lubben, & Kitano, 1989). Variation also exists within gender; more heavy drinking was seen among Japanese men (29%) than among Chinese men (14%) (Chi et al., 1989). Latinos exhibit variation in drinking related to a variety of sociocultural factors including gender and country of origin. Thus, among a randomly selected sample of Latinos living in the U.S., Mexican-American men (44%) tended to drink more heavily than Puerto Rican men (24%) and Cuban-American men (6%) (Caetano, 1989a). Although Mexican-American women drank more than other Latinas, their rates of heavy drinking were relatively low (14%) when compared to their male counterparts. In this sample, both income and education were positively related to drinking, particularly among males (Caetano, 1989a). Although representative national samples of Latinos provide a basis for making generalizations about drinking behavior, they are likely to conceal many other sources of variations in drinking behavior. Some researchers have focused on regional samples where particular groups of Latinos predominate: Mexican-Americans in the southwest (California, Arizona, Texas) or Latinos from the Caribbean (Cubans, Puerto Ricans) in the east. But even within these broadly defined regions, differences indicative of the impact of the local social norms and context occur. Thus, in a sample of Mexican-Americans living in California and Texas, the Californians reported a more accepting attitude towards drinking, more drunkenness, and more alcohol-related problems and than did the Texans (Caetano, 1989b).

Research on the prevalence of alcohol use provides data on which generalizations about group tendencies can be made. Consideration of even broad within group factors (e.g., region, tribal affiliation, country of origin) adds complexity. Thus, prevalence data provide important evidence that drinking behavior is related to a number of sociocultural factors. However, generalizations based on ethnicity and/or gender do not capture the complex variations in drinking behavior.

## Future Research on Prevalence

In prevalence research, as in other areas, there is a clear need for behavioral/objective definitions of the constructs being studied (e.g., heavy drinking, alcohol abuse) so that results can be compared both within and between groups (Lex, 1987; Weibel-Orlando, 1985). The failure to include variables that could explain variations in drinking has been described and must be reiterated as an important area for future research and model building. Caetano (1990) among others has called for the use of multifactorial models of the role of sociocultural factors in drinking to account for within group variations in drinking. This would provide the potential to explain findings currently presented only at the descriptive level. Clearly gender is a source of variation within most ethnic groups, but explanations of gender differences must include consideration of variations within gender. Longitudinal research on the etiology of alcohol use and abuse, which builds on these multifactorial models, would contribute significantly to our knowledge. For example, it would allow for examination of issues such as the role of national origin and acculturation in the drinking behavior of groups, such as Asian-Americans and Hispanic-Americans, who have histories of emigrating to the U.S. It also would assist in the tracking of changes in drinking behavior as individuals and/or groups experience changes in their social position or in other important sociocultural characteristics.

## OVERVIEW OF RESEARCH
## ON THE PREVENTION OF ALCOHOL ABUSE

Prevention of alcohol use/abuse encompasses a wide variety of theories, strategies, and populations. Since initial use of alcohol and other substances typically begins during adolescence, many primary prevention efforts are implemented among this age group in the schools. These programs contain interventions designed to change the individual's knowledge, attitudes, and behavior regarding alcohol and/or reduce risks related to psychological characteristics (e.g., increase self-esteem). In fact, there is accumulating evidence that the components of this type of prevention program may not be very important in the broader context of the sociocultural context in which adolescents function. For example, in a longitudinal (1-year) assessment of a prevention program for a predominantly European-American sample of high school students, the variables typically targeted in school-based prevention programs (e.g., knowledge, self-esteem) did not predict drinking-related behavior, once social and demographic variables (e.g., gender, parents, friends) had been accounted for (Mauss, Hopkins, Weisheit, & Kearney, 1988). The authors· concluded that "the variables targeted by our classroom prevention program turned out to be relatively unimportant, at least net of other variables in the students' lives, over which the classroom curriculum could not be expected to exert much (if any) influence" (p. 59). Similarly, in research with 1,147 American-Indian youngsters (mean age = 10.27 years), cumulative risk factor scores based on variables such as family and peer smoking, family relationship, cultural identification and religiosity were significantly related to lifetime use of alcohol and other substances (Moncher, Holden, & Trimble, 1990). These studies suggest that sociocultural factors such as SES, peer relations, and poor family relationships are important predictors of substance use among adolescents regardless of their ethnic background (also see Oetting & Beauvais, 1987a, 1987b; Rhodes & Jason, 1990).

Reviews of research on the primary prevention of alcohol use among adolescents in the general population have been uniformly negative in their appraisal of the efficacy of school-based programs (Bangert-Downs, 1988; Moskowitz, 1989; Tobler, 1986). Most such reviews find support for changes in knowledge and attitudes regarding alcohol use, but few changes in drinking behavior. Moskowitz has suggested that the most efficacious policies for alcohol prevention are: increasing alcohol taxes, enforcing drunk-driving laws, and raising the minimum legal drinking age to 21 years. These broad-based public policy interventions are likely to impact on all members of the society, including females and members of various ethnic groups. However, some groups exhibit patterns that may call for more targeted prevention efforts. For example, among African-Americans, the heaviest drinking is seen among middle-aged men and women, not among youth. Therefore, research on prevention efforts targeted to lessening alcohol abuse in this older population is essential.

Many prevention programs for non-European ethnic groups are targeted at adolescents who are characterized as being at "high risk" for substance use/abuse. The designation of risk status often is arbitrary and may include membership in particular ethnic groups and/or being from a low SES background (particularly living in economically disadvantaged urban neighborhoods). Although the social position of the samples is likely to impact on their risk status (Oetting & Beauvais, 1987b; Rhodes & Jason, 1990; Wallace & Bachman, 1991), little if any attention is given to the larger social arena in which the adolescents function. In some cases programs steeped in the middle class assumptions and values of the researchers are applied to students from disadvantaged backgrounds. Even programs that contain the appropriate emphasis on "cultural sensitivity" by incorporating language differences and peer leaders may overlook the important role of the broader social environment and instead focus on characteristics of the individual. Rhodes and Jason (1990) have described this tendency to ignore the impact of economic disadvantage as limiting us to seeing substance use and other deviant behaviors "as resulting from a deficit in the person rather than one possible response that any healthy, adequately functioning individual might have to the disordered or developmentally hazardous environmental circumstances he or she confronts" (p. 396). If substance use represents a response to a maladaptive, disadvantaged environment, then prevention efforts that ignore the factors that create and sustain such environments are likely to fail.

## Future Research on Prevention of Alcohol Abuse

Future research on prevention is likely to vary based on the particular model of prevention being espoused and by the issues faced by different groups. Comprehensive reviews of the limitations of alcohol prevention research to date as well as areas for future research have been presented elsewhere (e.g., Moskowitz, 1989; Institute of Medicine, 1989). Given the focus of this article, I will emphasize the role of sociocultural factors in the prevention research on ethnic populations and women. Public health and sociocultural models may be particularly relevant to prevention efforts among ethnic populations. May (1986) recommended that prevention efforts for American-Indians be organized around public health approaches to reducing alcohol-related mortality and morbidity such as changing alcohol related laws (e.g., removal of prohibition on alcohol on some reservations). Other approaches of relevance to this community include education, particularly for youth, where the dissemination of information is combined with skills training to enhance self-esteem and individual empowerment. Lastly, May describes a need for research on the effect of community based preventive education to reduce the levels of alcohol use as well as the adverse medical consequences of alcohol abuse, particularly among high risk subgroups such as pregnant women. Moncher et al. (1990) also have identified key issues in prevention as they apply to American-Indians. These issues also are highly relevant to prevention with other ethnic populations. The three key issues are: (1) the development and testing of theories based on etiological constructs that may explain variations in substance use; (2) development of a theoretically based risk assessment model for targeting adolescents at high risk for substance use as well as identifying protective factors; (3) the need to address issues around bicultural identity and the development of culturally sensitive programs.

Moskowitz (1989) espoused a sociocultural model which suggested that effective prevention efforts should focus on changing social norms regarding alcohol use, rather than on attempting to change individual attitudes and behavior. Research on strategies for changing social norms for alcohol use and on the efficacy of these approaches is essential, because some groups may have norms and/ or reasons for substance use that are different from those of the general population. For example, health warnings about the impact of smoking have successfully reduced smoking rates for the general population. However, young women continue to initiate smoking at high rates, possibly as a function of their belief in smoking as a means of controlling weight and the salience of weight control among their cohort (Collins, 1993). Similarly, during the past decade changes in social norms regarding the use of illicit substances have led to general reduction in the use of illicit drugs among high school seniors and college students. However, a comparable change in norms regarding alcohol use has not occurred and rates of alcohol use have been relatively stable in this population over the same time period (Johnson et al. 1992). Oetting and Beauvais (1987a, 1987b) also highlight the role of social norms in their research on the impact of peer associations on drug use. In their view, effective prevention must "eventually influence the choice of peers, the formation of peer clusters, and the development of strong sanctions against drugs in the peer cluster" (Oetting & Beauvais, 1987a,

p. 212). More research on the impact of social norms on alcohol use, particularly as they pertain to peer influences (cf. Brook, Brook, Gordon, Whiteman, & Cohen, 1990), alcohol use by females (Fillmore, 1987), and the role of acculturation (Gilbert, 1991) is likely to enhance knowledge concerning effective prevention strategies.

Some ethnic communities have attempted to change social norms about alcohol by mobilizing prevention efforts to counteract the special targeting of ethnic groups by those who manufacture and sell alcohol. Their efforts have included confronting alcohol advertising targeted to their constituents, boycotting liquor stores and alcohol manufacturers, protesting the marketing of new products targeted to specific ethnic groups, as well as questioning the impact of civic projects sponsored by alcohol manufacturers (Hacker, Collins, & Jacobson, 1987; Maxwell & Jacobson, 1989; McMahon & Taylor, 1990). Research is needed on the impact of these community generated prevention efforts. Such research would not only provide information on the efficacy of this approach to prevention, but could also provide ideas for innovative prevention strategies that could be applied to other groups in other settings. A community prevention approach also suggests that prevention programs may be more effectively mounted in settings where the populations being targeted are likely to congregate, such as the workplace (Nathan, 1984), churches (Prugh, 1986-87), and child-care agencies (Noel & McCrady, 1984).

Many prevention programs developed for the general population are likely to emphasize the values and biases of the numerically larger European based culture. Prevention programs that are sensitive to non-European cultural traditions are likely to enhance prevention efforts targeted to ethnic groups. Such programs should reflect the norms and traditions of the group(s) being targeted as well as current issues being faced by specific subgroups. Thus, prevention among American-Indians should reflect specific tribal traditions as well as the epidemiology of alcohol use for specific groups, so as to better target those at high risk. Prevention among Latinos should reflect issues such as the role of acculturation. For example, drinking among Mexican-American females increases as a function of acculturation (Gilbert, 1991). Thus Gilbert suggests that prevention efforts should be targeted at young Latinas who may be caught in a conflict between the norms for moderate alcohol use in the general population of the U.S. and Mexican cultural norms against women's drinking. These examples highlight the fact that research on the efficacy of culturally sensitive prevention programs must be based on detailed knowledge of the variety of sociocultural and alcohol-related issues that are encountered by different groups.

Enhanced understanding of etiological sociocultural factors for alcohol use/abuse also suggests areas for prevention. Such prevention should not only focus on drinking behavior per se, but in addition, direct attention to broader social issues. One example particularly relevant to women is the possible link between childhood sexual victimization and alcohol abuse. To the extent that this link is substantiated, then interventions to reduce the sexual victimization of female children might reduce rates of alcohol abuse among women as these cohorts of children grow older. Wallace and Bachman (1991) also acknowledge that effective prevention does not have to focus on substance use per se, but instead could confront broader etiological factors. They recommend that prevention efforts include social policies that confront the impact of socioeconomic disadvantage, enhance academic achievement and religious commitment, provide supervised activities for adolescents, and maintain stable (two parent) families.

Family influences have been cited in numerous studies of the etiology of alcohol/substance use in ethnic and nonethnic populations (e.g., Brook et al., 1990; Moncher et al., 1990; Rhodes & Jason, 1990). Family-based prevention efforts could focus on issues specific to alcohol/substance use or more generally on maintaining effective family functioning. Definitions of the family unit are likely to vary based on sociocultural factors. Thus, notions of "the family" should be broad enough to include siblings, parents and other relatives, as well as others who play a significant role in the individual's life (cf. Collins, 1990). Finally, research on family-based alcohol prevention could contribute to knowledge of factors related to resiliency in youngsters who do not succumb to social and environmental influences to use/abuse alcohol.

While not exhaustive, the research outlined here clearly indicates the variety of issues that need to be included in a sociocultural approach to prevention. Methodological and conceptually sound research framed within this perspective can offer insights into the development of effective alcohol abuse prevention for persons of all ages from a variety of backgrounds and social strata.

## OVERVIEW OF RESEARCH
## ON THE TREATMENT OF ALCOHOL ABUSE

In comparison to the general population, non-European ethnic groups (except for Asian-Americans) tend to be over-represented in alcohol treatment surveys (Gilbert & Cervantes, 1986; Lex, 1987). Thus, the recent Institute of Medicine (1990) report on alcoholism treatment summarized the state-of-the-art by acknowledging sources of variation within non-European ethnic groups (e.g., SES, acculturation, tribal identity) and then outlining areas of consensus. Most groups shared the problems of facing economic barriers to alcohol treatment (lack of health insurance, reliance on public funding) and the lack of ethnically-oriented programs that exhibit cultural sensitivity. The report concluded by decrying the descriptive nature (mostly surveys) of the current alcohol treatment literature and the lack of studies on the relative efficacy of ethnically-oriented treatment approaches.

Among the issues found in treatment research on many ethnic groups are the limitations on the samples that are studied. For example, although African-Americans seeking alcoholism treatment are heterogeneous with regard to SES, age, and gender, the research tends to focus on lower SES, urban, male populations (Lex, 1987). This emphasis is not representative of the population and has overlooked issues faced by other subgroups of African-Americans, particularly African-American women. When these issues are examined, within group differences may become apparent. For example, gender differences in treatment participation by African-Americans were found in a sample of low SES (53% unemployed, 53% had not completed high school), middle-aged men and women in a "culturally sensitive" treatment program (Burlew, Butler, Lewis, & Washington, 1992). Specifically, females were less likely to complete treatment than males (45% and 67%, respectively) and they attended fewer individual and group therapy sessions than did their male counterparts. These findings indicate that even when culturally appropriate treatment was available, African-American women were less responsive to treatment than were their male counterparts. If such is the case, then treatment research on African-Americans must include appropriate samples of women as well as consideration of other important sociocultural factors that may impact on treatment outcome.

Gilbert and Cervantes (1986) have published one of the few reviews of alcoholism treatment among Mexican-Americans. Citing numerous limitations in gaining access to utilization figures (e.g., differential coding across states and years), they focus on the five southwestern states where Mexican-Americans predominate (Arizona, California, Colorado, New Mexico, and Texas). Data for four of the five states indicated that Mexican-American adults were over-represented (only Arizona showed under-utilization) in alcoholism treatment. Most of this over-representation occurred because of the alcohol problems of Mexican-American males. Their female counterparts were significantly under-represented in alcoholism treatment. These male alcoholics tended to be married and employed, suggesting greater social and economic stability. They were more likely to be involved in outpatient treatment rather than either detoxification or inpatient treatment. Possibly related to their greater stability, Mexican-American males were seen as good candidates for achieving successful treatment outcomes (Gilbert & Cervantes, 1986).

Although American-Indians represent some 1% of the U.S. population, they are said to represent 6% of those in alcoholism treatment (Lex 1987). Some 28% of those in treatment are women and many of those in treatment are of lower SES (unemployed, low income), unmarried, and in need of inpatient care. Treatment outcomes among American-Indians have tended to be poor (Lex 1987). One of the few systematic assessments of American-Indian response to treatment was undertaken in the state of Washington (Walker, Benjamin, Kivlahan, & Walker, 1989). The predominantly male sample of chronic alcoholics represented "39 tribes and 10 cultural groups . . ." (p. 303), was from low SES backgrounds, and was socially unstable (poor, unemployed, mobile, no family support). They were followed for up to 2 years. Fifty of the subjects were primarily involved in detoxification, but also participated in halfway houses and some inpatient treatment. Only three of these subjects reported a significant period (6 months) of abstinence. The majority (over 84% of a sample of 90) of those involved in inpatient and halfway house treatment continued to abuse alcohol. Generally treatment was not effective for this sample, and even an Indian-specific treatment program was no more effective than an integrated program. However, given the possible role of social disadvantage in the etiology of substance use among American-Indians (cf. Wallace & Bachman, 1991), it is not surprising that traditional treatment approaches, even a program containing culturally relevant components, were not successful.

Treatment research on non-European ethnic groups and women is in its infancy, and as such, findings are limited. The research to date clearly indicates the existence of within group differences and the impact of sociocultural factors such as economic status. It also indicates that treatment outcome for women and members of ethnic groups is relatively poor. Although this assessment occurs within the context of the generally poor outcome for alcoholism treatment, regardless of ethnicity or gender (Institute of Medicine, 1990), it suggests the need for innovation in designing and conducting treatment research that includes sociocultural factors.

## RECOMMENDATIONS FOR FUTURE RESEARCH ON TREATMENT FOR ALCOHOL ABUSE

Given the paucity of research on the impact of sociocultural factors in treatment, research on almost any topic would enhance knowledge that may be relevant to gender, ethnicity, and/or subgroups within particular ethnic designations. As researchers and policy makers have become more aware of major gaps in knowledge, recommendations for improvements in treatment research have come from a number of quarters. While methodological critiques and recommendations are not the focus of the following section, it is hoped that future research conducted on topics related to the role of sociocultural factors will employ state-of-the-art methodologies in research design, scale development, and statistical analyses.

Sociocultural factors are likely to have an impact on various aspects of treatment, ranging from availability (which is often related to SES) to treatment outcome. Many of the recommendations for future research on treatment are based on those characteristics that may be related to improved outcome among women and ethnic populations. One clear need for the future is basic information on treatment availability, admission and referral practices, drop out rates, and relapse rates as they relate to SES (which is related to access to treatment and treatment outcome) as well as gender, ethnicity and other sociocultural factors (cf. Gilbert & Cervantes, 1986). For example, women, African-Americans, and Hispanics are less likely to complete outpatient alcohol treatment (Mammo & Weinbaum, 1993), and some of the reasons for this may relate to the failure to acknowledge sociocultural factors in the design and implementation of treatment programs. It is possible that more broadly conceived community-oriented treatment programs that include interventions to enhance life adjustment (e.g., finding a job, improve social relationships) would enhance treatment completion (and outcome) among disadvantaged problem drinkers (cf. Azrin, 1976; Hunt & Azrin, 1973).

There have been many acknowledgments of cultural barriers to treatment and related calls for culturally-sensitive treatment. Dependent on group, such treatment could involve bilingual-bicultural staff (Caste & Blodgett, 1979; Gilbert & Cervantes, 1986; Institute of Medicine, 1990), traditional healing, or a focus on religion and various spiritual practices (Caste & Blodgett, 1979; May, 1986; Prugh, 1986-87; Weibel-Orlando, 1985), as well as sensitivity to historical and economic circumstances that impact on drinking behavior (Herd, 1985; Lex, 1987; Weibel-Orlando, 1986-87). Many obvious questions exist about the inclusion of culturally sensitive material into alcoholism treatment. For example, must culturally sensitive treatment involve separation into ethnic and/or gender based groups, as is often recommended (Burlew et al., 1992; Gilbert & Cervantes, 1986; Institute of Medicine, 1990)? Can culturally-relevant materials be added to existing treatment packages or must new treatment strategies be developed based on the sociocultural characteristics of different populations? Does a match between the sociocultural characteristics of treatment providers and clients enhance the efficacy of culturally sensitive treatment? These questions represent only a beginning to considering culturally sensitive approaches to alcohol treatment. Recommendations to conduct comparative outcome studies on the efficacy of specific treatment techniques as applied to different groups are quite common (Gilbert & Cervantes, 1986; Institute of Medicine, 1990). This issue must be approached with caution because unless there are theoretical reasons for assuming that ethnicity (or gender) would produce differential responses to particular techniques, then such studies are less likely to be necessary. For example, behavioral treatment techniques that focus on the acquisition of specific skills may be neutral with regard to both gender and ethnicity. In fact, it has been suggested that behavioral treatment that includes moderation goals may be very appropriate given the cultural context of some ethnic groups (Bach & Bornstein, 1981). Similarly, when compared to men, women have shown a greater ability to drink moderately after behavioral treatment (Helzer et al., 1985; Miller & Joyce, 1979; Sanchez-Craig, Leigh, Spivak, & Lei, 1989), suggesting that women may be excellent candidates for behavioral interventions.

At this time we have few indicators of what techniques from what theoretical orientations are likely to produce different and/or better outcomes based on the sociocultural characteristics of participants in treatment. As a likely consequence of the heterogeneity within groups, there are few consistent patterns of response to alcoholism treatment based on ethnicity. Similarly, reviews of treatment outcome in which men and women are treated similarly have shown inconsistent results concerning the impact of gender (Collins, 1993). Thus, dependent on the nature and/or form of treatment as well as the populations being examined, comparative studies of ethnic or gender based groupings may or may not be useful. However, studies that consider sources of variation within groups are likely to add to knowledge. All such studies should include long term follow-ups (12 months or longer) of treatment efficacy.

One area in which sociocultural factors are likely to play an important role is family treatment for alcohol problems. Sociocultural differences among ethnic groups are likely to include different family structures, norms, and expectations regarding family roles. For example, family-oriented interventions, particularly the provision of support for nonalcoholic partners and extended family, have been recommended for Mexican-American alcoholics, who as a group tend to be socially stable and come from a family-centered culture (Gilbert & Cervantes, 1986). Since aspects of Mexican-American culture may create complex dynamics around family and alcohol use (Caetano, 1986-87), this seems an area ripe for research. Other ethnic groups also possess sociocultural characteristics that may make them good candidates for family interventions, if such interventions are tailored to meet the characteristics of the group. Similarly, the different gender and life roles of men and women are likely to impact on various aspects of the response to family treatment (Collins, 1990). Even so, little or no attention has been given to ethnic or gender variations in research on family-oriented alcoholism treatment.

## CONCLUSIONS

The state-of-the-art for research on sociocultural factors as they pertain to ethnicity and gender is not good. The research reviewed here suggests limited conceptual and methodological progress in this area of research. However, the recommendations contained in this review suggest many fruitful areas for future research. There are some rays of hope that these recommendations could be realized. The current mandate to include women and under-represented ethnic groups in federally funded research has the potential to increase progress in these areas. However, this potential can only be realized if researchers adopt new approaches to conceptual and methodological issues related to conducting research with ethnic samples and with women. Research that conforms to the words of the federal guidelines by relying on ethnic glosses or gender-based stereotypes will not add to knowledge and may end up reifying the status quo. It is not sufficient to include a low income African-American sample of adolescents in a prevention study if the strategies being tested are not informed by knowledge of the range of social and cultural issues faced by these adolescents. It is not sufficient to include women in a treatment outcome study if the treatment strategies do not address issues unique to female alcoholics. Although the researcher does not have to possess the demographic or sociocultural characteristics of the population being studied, the successful researcher is likely to be one who is open to understanding the impact of these characteristics and to contributing not only to scientific knowledge but also to the individuals and communities in which they conduct research. One potential area for making significant contributions is in the training and mentoring of researchers who are female or from non-European backgrounds. The pool of researchers that could be developed as a result of such efforts is likely to ensure future progress in all areas of research on alcohol use and abuse.

## REFERENCES

Azrin, N. H. (1976). Improvements in the community reinforcement approach to alcoholism. *Behaviour Research and Therapy, 14*, 339-348.

Bach, P. J., & Bornstein, P. H. (1981). A social learning rationale and suggestions for behavioral treatment with American Indian alcohol abusers. *Addictive Behaviors, 6*, 75-81.

Bangert-Drowns, R. L. (1988). The effects of school-based substance abuse education: A meta-analysis. *Journal of Drug Education, 18*, 243-264.

Beckman, L. J., & Amaro, H. (1986). Personal and social difficulties faced by women and men entering alcoholism treatment. *Journal of Studies on Alcohol, 47*, 135-145.

Brook, J. S., Brook, D. W., Gordon, A. S., Whiteman, M., & Cohen, P. (1990). The psychosocial etiology of adolescent drug use: A family interactional approach. *Genetic, Social, and General Psychology Monographs, 116*, 111-267.

Burlew, A. K. H., Butler, J., Lewis, N., & Washington, K. (1992). Gender differences in the participation of African-Americans in alcoholism treatment. In A. K. H. Burlew, W. C. Banks, H. P. McAdoo, & D. A. Azibo (Eds.), *African American psychology: Theory, research, and practice* (pp. 346-355). Newbury Park: Sage Publications.

Caetano, R. (1986). Alternative definitions of Hispanics: Consequences in an alcohol survey. *Hispanic Journal of Behavioral Sciences, 8*, 331-344.

Caetano, R. (1986-87). Drinking and Hispanic-American family life: The view outside the clinic walls. *Alcohol Health & Research World, 11*, 26-33.

Caetano, R. (1989a). Drinking patterns and alcohol problems in a national sample of U. S. Hispanics. In D. Spiegler, D. Tate, S. Aitken, & C. Christian (Eds.), *Alcohol use among U. S. ethnic minorities* (pp. 147-162; DHHS Publication No. (ADM) 89-1435). Washington, DC: U.S. Government Printing Office.

Caetano, R. (1989b). Differences in alcohol use between Mexican Americans in Texas and California. *Hispanic Journal of Behavioral Sciences, 11*, 58-69.

Caetano, R. (1990). Hispanic drinking in the US: Thinking in new directions. *British Journal of Addiction, 85*, 1231-1236.

Caste, C. A., & Blodgett, J. W. (1979). Cultural barriers in the utilization of alcohol programs by Hispanics in the United States. In J. Szapocznik (Ed.), *Mental health, drug and alcohol abuse: An Hispanic assessment of present and future challenges* (pp. 61-70). Washington, DC: National Coalition of Hispanic Mental Health and Human Services Organizations.

Cheung, Y. W. (1989). Making sense of ethnicity and drug use: A review and suggestions for future research. *Social Pharmacology, 3*, 55-82.

Chi, I., Lubben, J. E., & Kitano, H. H. L. (1989). Differences in drinking behavior among three Asian-American groups. *Journal of Studies on Alcohol, 50*, 15-23.

Chomak, S., & Collins, R. L. (1987). Relationship between sex-role behaviors and alcohol consumption in undergraduate men and women. *Journal of Studies on Alcohol, 48*, 194-201.

Christian, C. M., Zobeck, T. S., Malin, H. J., & Hitchcock, D. C. (1989). Self-reported alcohol use and abuse among Mexican Americans: Preliminary findings from the Hispanic Health and Nutrition Examination Survey adult sample person supplement. In D. Spiegler, D. Tate, S. Aitken, & C. Christian (Eds.), *Alcohol use among U. S. ethnic minorities* (pp. 425-438; DHHS Publication No. (ADM) 89-1435). Washington, DC: U.S. Government Printing Office.

Collins, R. L. (1990). Family treatment of alcohol abuse: Behavioral and systems perspectives. In R. L. Collins, K. E. Leonard, & J. S. Searles (Eds.), *Alcohol and the family: Research and clinical perspectives* (pp. 285-308). New York: Guilford.

Collins, R. L. (1992). Methodological issues in conducting substance abuse research on ethnic minority populations. *Drugs & Society, 6*, 59-77.

Collins, R. L. (1993). Women's issues in alcohol use and cigarette smoking. In J. S. Baer, G. A. Marlatt, & R. J. McMahon (Eds.), *Addictive behaviors across the lifespan: Prevention, treatment, and policy issues* (pp. 274-306). Newbury Park, CA: Sage.

Colliver, J., Grigson, M. B., Barbano, H., Dufour, M., & Malin, H. (1989). NHANES I epidemiologic follow up study: Methodological issues and preliminary findings. In D. Spiegler, D. Tate, S. Aitken, & C. Christian (Eds.), *Alcohol use among U. S. ethnic minorities* (pp. 411-423; DHHS Publication No. (ADM) 89-1435). Washington, DC: U.S. Government Printing Office.

Critchlow, B. (1986). The powers of John Barleycorn: Beliefs about the effects of alcohol on social behavior. *American Psychologist, 41*, 751-764.

Dawson, D. A., & Archer, L. (1992). Gender differences in alcohol consumption: Effects of measurement. *British Journal of Addiction, 87*, 119-123.

Fillmore, K. M. (1987). Women's drinking across the adult life course as compared to men. *British Journal of Addiction, 82*, 801-811.

Fisher, A. D. (1987). Alcoholism and race: The misapplication of both concepts to North American Indians. *The Canadian Review of Sociology and Anthropology, 24*, 81-98.

Gilbert, M. J. (1991). Acculturation and changes in drinking patterns among

Mexican-American women: Implications for prevention. *Alcohol Health & Research World, 15*, 234-238.

Gilbert, M. J., & Cervantes, R. C. (1986). Alcohol services for Mexican Americans: A review of utilization patterns, treatment considerations and prevention activities. *Hispanic Journal of Behavioral Sciences, 8*, 191-223.

Gilbert, M. J., & Collins, R. L. (in press). Ethnic variation in women and men's drinking. In R. W. Wilsnack & S. C. Wilsnack (Eds.), *Gender and alcohol.* Piscataway, NJ: Rutgers Center of Alcohol Studies.

Hacker, G. A., Collins, R., & Jacobson, M. (1987). *Marketing booze to Blacks.* Washington, DC: Center for Science in the Public Interest.

Heath, D. B. (1990-91). Uses and misuses of the concept of ethnicity in alcohol studies: An essay in deconstruction. *The International Journal of the Addictions, 25*, 607-628.

Helzer, J. E., Robins, L. N., Taylor, J. R., Carey, K., Miller, R. H., Combs-Orme, T., & Farmer, A. (1985). The extent of long-term moderate drinking among alcoholics discharged from medical and psychiatric treatment facilities. *New England Journal of Medicine, 312*, 1678-1682.

Herd, D. (1985). Ambiguity in black drinking norms. An ethnohistorical interpretation. In L. A. Bennett & G. M. Ames (Eds.), *The American experience with alcohol: Contrasting cultural perspectives* (pp. 149-170). New York: Plenum Press.

Herd, D. (1989). The epidemiology of drinking patterns and alcohol-related problems among U. S. Blacks. In D. Spiegler, D. Tate, S. Aitken, & C. Christian (Eds.), *Alcohol use among U.S ethnic minorities* (pp. 3-50; DHHS Publication No. (ADM) 89-1435). Washington, DC: U.S. Government Printing Office.

Hilton, M. E. (1987). Drinking patterns and drinking problems in 1984: Results from a general population survey. *Alcoholism: Clinical and Experimental Research, 11*, 167-174.

Hunt, G. M., & Azrin, N. H. (1973). A community reinforcement approach to alcoholism. *Behaviour Research and Therapy, 11*, 91-104.

Hurley, D. L. (1991). Women, alcohol and incest: An analytical review. *Journal of Studies on Alcohol, 52*, 253-268.

Institute of Medicine (1989). *Prevention and treatment of alcohol problems: Research opportunities.* Washington, DC: National Academy Press.

Institute of Medicine (1990). *Broadening the base of treatment for alcohol problems.* Washington, DC: National Academy Press.

Johnson, L. D., O'Malley, P. M., & Bachman, J. G. (1992). *Smoking, drinking, and illicit drug use among American secondary school students, college students, and young adults, 1975-1991.* Rockville, MD: National Institute on Drug Abuse.

Leland, J. (1984). Alcohol use and abuse in ethnic minority women: "Different strokes for different folks." In S. C. Wilsnack & L. J. Beckman (Eds.), *Alcohol problems in women* (pp. 66-96). New York: Guilford.

Lex, B. W. (1987). Review of alcohol problems in ethnic minority groups. *Journal of Consulting and Clinical Psychology, 55*, 293-300.

Lex, B. W. (1991). Some gender differences in alcohol and polysubstance users. *Health Psychology, 10*, 121-132.

Lubben, J. E., Chi, I., & Kitano, H. H. L. (1988). Exploring Filipino American drinking behavior. *Journal of Studies on Alcohol, 49*, 26-29.

MacAndrew, C., & Edgerton, R. B. (1969). Drunken comportment: A social explanation. New York: Aldine.

Mammo, A., & Weinbaum, D. F. (1993). Some factors that influence dropping out from outpatient alcoholism treatment facilities. *Journal of Studies on Alcohol, 54*, 92-101.

Marlatt, G. A., & Rohsenow, D. J. (1980). Cognitive processes in alcohol use: Expectancy and the balanced placebo design. In N. K. Mello (Ed.), *Advances in substance abuse, Vol. 1* (pp. 159-199). Greenwich, CT: JAI Press.

Mauss, A. L., Hopkins, R. H., Weisheit, R. A., & Kearney, K. A. (1988). The problematic prospects for prevention in the classroom: Should alcohol education programs be expected to reduce drinking by youth? *Journal of Studies on Alcohol, 49*, 51-61.

Maxwell, B., & Jacobson, M. (1989). *Marketing disease to Hispanics: The selling of alcohol, tobacco, and junk foods.* Washington, DC: Center for Science in the Public Interest.

May, P. A. (1986). Alcohol and drug misuse prevention programs for American Indians: Needs and opportunities. *Journal of Studies on Alcohol, 47*, 187-195.

May, P. A., & Smith, M. B. (1988). Some Navajo Indian options about alcohol abuse and prohibition: A survey and recommendations for policy. *Journal of Studies on Alcohol, 49*, 324-334.

McMahon, E. T., & Taylor, P. A. (1990). *Citizens' action handbook on alcohol and tobacco billboard advertising.* Washington, DC: Center for Science in the Public Interest.

Midanik, L. T., & Room, R. (1992). The epidemiology of alcohol consumption. *Alcohol Health & Research World, 16*, 183-190.

Miller, B. A., Downs, W. R., Gondoli, D. M., & Keil, A. (1987). The role of childhood sexual abuse in the development of alcoholism in women. *Violence and Victims, 2*, 157-172.

Miller, W. R., & Joyce, M. A. (1979). Prediction of abstinence, controlled drinking, and heavy drinking outcomes following behavioral self-control training. *Journal of Consulting and Clinical Psychology, 47*, 773-775.

Moncher, M. S., Holden, G. W., & Trimble, J. E. (1990). Substance abuse among Native-American youth. *Journal of Consulting and Clinical Psychology, 58*, 408-415.

Moskowitz, J. M. (1989). The primary prevention of alcohol problems: A critical review of the research literature. *Journal of Studies on Alcohol, 50*, 54-88.

Nathan, P. E. (1984). Alcoholism prevention in the workplace: Three examples. In P. M. Miller & T. D. Nirenberg (Eds.), *Prevention of alcohol abuse* (pp. 387-405). New York: Plenum Press.

National Institute on Alcohol Abuse and Alcoholism. (1990). *Seventh special* report to the U.S. Congress on alcohol and health. (DHHS Publication No. (ADM) 90-1656). Washington DC: U. S. Government Printing Office.

Noel, N. E., & McCrady, B. S. (1984). Target populations for alcohol abuse prevention. In P. M. Miller & T. D. Nirenberg (Eds.), Prevention of alcohol abuse (pp. 55-94). New York: Plenum Press.

Oetting, E. R., & Beauvais, F. (1987a). Peer cluster theory, socialization characteristics, and adolescent drug use: A path analysis. Journal of Counseling Psychology, 34, 205-213.

Oetting, E. R., & Beauvais, F. (1987b). Common elements in youth drug abuse: Peer clusters and other psychosocial factors. Journal of Drug Issues, 17, 133-151.

Oetting, E. R., & Beauvais, F. (1990-91). Orthogonal cultural identification theory: The cultural identification of minority adolescents. The International Journal of the Addictions, 25, 655-685.

Osborne, N. G., & Feit, M. D. (1992). The use of race in medical research. Journal of the American Medical Association, 267, 275-279.

Prugh, T. (1986-87). The Black church: A foundation for recovery. Alcohol Health & Research World, 11, 52-55.

Rhodes, J. E., & Jason, L. A. (1990). A social stress model of substance abuse. Journal of Consulting and Clinical Psychology, 58, 395-401.

Sanchez-Craig, M., Leigh, G., Spivak, K., & Lei, H. (1989). Superior outcome of females over males after brief treatment for the reduction of heavy drinking. British Journal of Addiction, 84, 395-404.

Thom, B. (1986). Sex differences in help-seeking for alcohol problems: I. The barriers to help seeking. British Journal of Addiction, 81, 777-788.

Tobler, N. S. (1986). Meta-analysis of 143 adolescent drug prevention programs: Quantitative outcome results of program participants compared to a control or comparison group. Journal of Drug Issues, 16, 537-567.

Trimble, J. E. (1990-91). Ethnic specification, validation prospect, and the future of drug use research. International Journal of the Addictions, 25, 149-170.

Walker, R. D., Benjamin, G. A., Kivlahan, D., & Walker, P. S. (1989). American Indian alcohol misuse and treatment outcome. In D. Spiegler, D. Tate, S. Aitken, & C. Christian (Eds.), Alcohol use among U. S. ethnic minorities (411-423; DHHS Publication No. (ADM) 89-1435). Washington, DC: U.S. Government Printing Office.

Wallace, J. M., & Bachman, J. G. (1991). Explaining racial/ethnic differences in adolescent drug use: The impact of background and lifestyle. Social Problems, 38, 333-357.

Weibel-Orlando, J. C. (1985). Indians, ethnicity, and alcohol. Contrasting perceptions of the ethnic self and alcohol use. In L. A. Bennett & G. M. Ames (Eds.), The American experience with alcohol: Contrasting cultural perspectives (pp. 201-226). New York: Plenum Press.

Weibel-Orlando, J. C. (1986-87). Drinking patterns of urban and rural American Indians. Alcohol Health & Research World, 11, 8-12.

Weibel-Orlando, J. C. (1989). Pass the bottle, Bro!: A comparison of urban and rural Indian drinking patterns. In D. Spiegler, D. Tate, S. Aitken, & C. Christian (Eds.), *Alcohol use among U.S ethnic minorities* (pp. 259-289; DHHS Publication No. (ADM) 89-1435). Washington, DC: U.S. Government Printing Office.

Wilsnack, S. C., Wilsnack, R. W., & Klassen, A. D. (1985). Drinking and drinking problems among women in a U.S. national survey. *Alcohol Health & Research World, 9,* 3-13.

Wilson, G. T. (1988). Alcohol use and abuse: A social learning analysis. In C. D. Chaudron & D. A. Wilkinson (Eds.), *Theories on alcoholism* (pp. 239-287). Toronto: Addiction Research Foundation.

# Drinking Moderation Training as a Contemporary Therapeutic Approach

## Gerard J. Connors

**SUMMARY.** Research on moderate drinking treatments, while remaining controversial in the United States, has extended our knowledge regarding alcohol use disorders and raised important theoretical and practical issues to be addressed in future research. The present assessment of the current status of drinking moderation treatments focuses on two topics. The first concerns the viability of moderate drinking treatment approaches as a contemporary therapeutic strategy. The second topic is whether research on moderate drinking has helped or hindered progress in the treatment of alcohol problems. It is argued that moderate drinking techniques indeed are a viable treatment approach for some alcohol abusers and that research in this area has fostered progress in the treatment of alcohol problems. Some directions for future research are identified.

Gerard J. Connors is a senior research scientist at the Research Institute on Addictions, Buffalo, NY 14203.

The author would like to thank the following colleagues for their valued and insightful comments on an earlier draft of this manuscript: Howard T. Blane, R. Lorraine Collins, Stephen A. Maisto, Linda C. Sobell, and Kimberly S. Walitzer. However, the comments and opinions presented in this article should be viewed as those only of the author.

Preparation of this manuscript was supported in part by Grant AA08076 from the National Institute on Alcohol Abuse and Alcoholism.

[Haworth co-indexing entry note]: "Drinking Moderation Training as a Contemporary Therapeutic Approach," Connors, Gerard J. Co-published simultaneously in *Drugs & Society* (The Haworth Press, Inc.) Vol. 8, No. 1, 1993, pp. 117-134; and: *Innovations in Alcoholism Treatment: State of the Art Reviews and Their Implications for Clinical Practice* (ed: Gerard J. Connors) The Haworth Press, Inc., 1993, pp. 117-134. Multiple copies of this article/chapter may be purchased from The Haworth Document Delivery Center [1-800-3-HAWORTH; 9:00 a.m. - 5:00 p.m. (EST)].

*117*

## INTRODUCTION

The past two decades have been characterized by a remarkable growth in research on alcohol problems, including but not limited to research in the areas of the biology and biochemistry, genetics, epidemiology, psychological factors, and prevention and treatment (NIAAA, 1990). Advances in all of these domains have expanded our knowledge regarding alcohol use and abuse and raised important theoretical and practical issues to be addressed in future research.

Such is the case with research on moderate (or "controlled") drinking, the topic of the present article. This paper focuses on drinking moderation as a contemporary therapeutic approach in the treatment of alcohol use disorders. The article is divided into several sections. The first section provides an overview of some of the historical highlights that have transpired in this area over the past decades. Following the historical overview will be an assessment of the current status of moderate drinking approaches. This assessment will concentrate on two issues. The first is whether moderate drinking training is a viable contemporary therapeutic approach in the treatment of alcohol use disorders. The second issue contemplated is whether research on moderate drinking has helped or hindered the advancement of treatment of alcohol problems. The subsequent section will identify some directions for future research in this area, and the article closes with several general conclusions on moderate drinking treatments.

## HISTORICAL OVERVIEW

Posttreatment moderate drinking among persons treated for alcohol use disorders is not a novel outcome or proposition. Clinical researchers for many years have identified subgroups of alcoholics treated for alcoholism who have demonstrated a pattern of drinking without problems or indications of dependence on alcohol following treatment. Examples of such outcomes have been reported since at least the 1940s, frequently as part of follow-up studies. A representative follow-up study was reported by Selzer and Holloway

(1957). They assessed the posttreatment drinking of 98 alcoholics 6-7 years after being hospitalized for treatment of alcoholism. Among 83 patients for whom sufficient data were available to assess adjustment, 18 (22%) became abstinent and 16 (19%) became moderate drinkers. Forty-one of the clients thus were classified as "essentially rehabilitated" (p. 118). The 16 classified as moderate drinkers represented 14 of the 59 males (24%) evaluated and 2 of the 24 (8%) females. Selzer and Holloway (1957) described this group as follows:

> [This group] comprised 16 patients of whom 12 continued to drink smaller amounts of alcohol than previously and 4 drank somewhat less and at much longer intervals than in the past. All 16 of these patients made a definitely adequate posthospital adjustment. This group later acquired a seventeenth member who in 1953, after years of alcoholism, became a moderate drinker. Thus apparently 12 of these patients (later 13) became social drinkers despite a number of years during which they were unquestionably alcoholics. (p. 114)

Selzer and Holloway (1957) later stated that "The fact that 16 per cent of 83 patients were able to return to social or nonpathological drinking, seems to warrant a second look at the long-cherished theory that no alcoholic can ever become a moderate drinker" (p. 114-115).

Such outcomes apparently were taken in stride by some investigators, since Selzer and Holloway combined these clients with the abstinent clients to comprise an "essentially rehabilitated" group. As noted by Miller (1983), this suggests that positive treatment outcomes were conceptualized to some extent simply as the *remission* of drinking problems, as opposed to the achievement of total abstinence. However, such outcomes could then, as now, be controversial. Selzer (1963), in later describing the presentation of these data, reported that the findings "prompted the agency that provided funds for the study virtually to order us to omit these 'embarrassing' findings" (p. 113).

Despite reports of moderate drinking outcomes over a period of years, the publication of similar outcomes by Davies (1962) in the *Quarterly Journal of Studies on Alcohol* elicited a much different response, perhaps because his article focused solely on these drinkers. Davies (1962) obtained drinking outcome data from 93 alcoholics hospitalized and treated 7-11 years earlier for alcoholism. He found at follow-up that seven (7.5%) of these patients (all male) had been engaged in nonproblematic moderate drinking after treatment and provided profiles of them. It is noteworthy that Davies (1962) perceived these patients to be a minority subgroup of alcoholics. In fact, he closed his article by stating that "It is not denied that the majority of alcohol addicts are incapable of achieving 'normal drinking.' All patients should be told to aim at total abstinence" (p. 103).

The reaction to Davies' descriptions of these seven patients was robust. A host of responding comments appeared in the *Quarterly Journal of Studies on Alcohol* over the following year (see Block, 1962; Lemere, 1963; Lolli, 1963; Myerson, 1963; Selzer, 1963; and Tiebout, 1962, for a sampling of these responses). A recurrent theme in the comments was the dismissal of the findings as having little clinical significance (Edwards, 1985a, and Roizen, 1987, have provided detailed evaluations of the responses). Others in the years since have suggested that the Davies report set in place the groundwork for subsequent paradigmatic changes in conceptualizing alcohol problems (e.g., Edwards, 1985a; Heather & Robertson, 1981; Pattison, 1976). Regardless of the validity of this proposition, the Davies (1962) article, notwithstanding a qualifying report on these clients by Edwards (1985b), remains a milestone in the recognition of and thinking about moderate drinking outcomes among persons with alcohol problems.

The topic of moderate drinking did not resurface again in any controversial manner in the 1960s, although research on and reviews of the topic did appear (e.g., Pattison, 1966; Pattison, Headley, Gleser, & Gottschalk, 1968; Reinert & Bowen, 1968). Additional controversy arose in the 1970s. Most noteworthy among the 1970s events were clinical outcome studies by Lovibond and Caddy (1970) and Sobell and Sobell (1973a, 1973b, 1976), laboratory studies on alcohol use and alcohol effects (summarized by Heather and Robertson, 1981), and the Rand Reports (Armor, Polich, & Stambul, 1978; Polich, Armor, & Braiker, 1981).

The Lovibond and Caddy (1970) and Sobell and Sobell (1973a,

1973b, 1976) studies are of particular importance because they are among the earliest to empirically evaluate moderate drinking as a specific treatment objective. Lovibond and Caddy (1970) studied the effects of a treatment that included training in blood alcohol level discrimination, the administration of shocks when alcohol concentrations exceeded a particular level during conditioning sessions, family member involvement, and self-control counseling. Twenty-one of 28 alcoholics receiving this treatment were classified as successful moderate drinkers at follow-up points ranging from 16-60 weeks. A comparison group, which received an identical treatment except that noncontingent shocks were administered during conditioning sessions, did not do as well.

The Sobell and Sobell (1973a, 1973b, 1976) study is better known to many in the alcohol field, and will be reviewed here only briefly. In their study, male alcoholics entering hospital treatment for alcoholism were first evaluated for suitability for either a moderate drinking or abstinent treatment goal. Patients seen as appropriate for a treatment goal of moderate drinking were assigned randomly to receive either a treatment focused on developing moderate drinking skills or to a control group that received the hospital's existing treatment focused on abstinence. Patients evaluated as appropriate for an abstinence-oriented treatment goal were randomly assigned to either a behaviorally-oriented treatment focused on abstinence or to a control group that received the hospital's existing abstinence-based treatment. The major finding regarding moderate drinking treatment was that the patients who received moderate drinking training were functioning significantly better at the one- and two-year follow-ups than the moderate drinking-eligible patients who received the abstinence-based treatment (Sobell & Sobell, 1973b, 1976). These outcomes were replicated in an independent third-year follow-up of these patients (Caddy, Addington, & Perkins, 1978).

The Sobell and Sobell (1973a, 1973b, 1976) reports on training moderate drinking skills had a major influence in the scientific community, but did not elicit at that time the widespread response previously accorded the Davies (1962) report or later accorded the Rand Reports (Armor et al., 1978; Polich et al., 1981) or the Pendery, Maltzman, and West (1982) report on the moderate drinking patients from the Sobell and Sobell study.

Also occurring in the 1970s was controlled research on drinking behavior and alcohol effects among alcoholics, represented by Cohen, Liebson, and Faillace (1972), Cohen, Liebson, Faillace, and Speers (1971), Engle and Williams (1972), and Mello and Mendelson (1972). This laboratory research has been reviewed in detail by Heather and Robertson (1981, pp. 78-129). Pertinent to the present discussion is that much of this research showed that severely dependent alcoholics were able to consume alcohol without exhibiting loss of control drinking or craving. Such findings, especially the observation that alcoholics in controlled environments could drink moderately, provided an empirical and theoretical foundation for later efforts to train alcoholics to drink in moderation.

The Rand Reports, appearing later in the 1970s, described the posttreatment functioning of clients seeking clinical services for drinking problems at alcoholism treatment centers across the nation. The first Rand Report (Armor et al., 1978) described 18-month follow-up data and the second (Polich et al., 1981) described four-year outcome data. The first report aroused much controversy because of the finding that some of the patients treated (22%) were engaged in normal drinking at 18-month follow-up. The second report, in addition to incorporating four-year outcome data, attempted to address methodological concerns with the 18-month follow-up (e.g., representativeness of the sample, attrition, validity of the self-reports, criteria for normal drinking, and use of a brief window in assessing outcome; see Armor, Stambul, & Polich, 1977; Blume, 1977; Emrick & Stilson, 1977; Smith & Jackson, 1982). In the second Rand Report, which received less fanfare than the first, there existed a group of clients (18%) who were engaged in moderate drinking without problems or indications of dependence. These outcomes occurred in the absence of treatments geared toward moderate drinking. In addition, only 7% of the sample had been abstinent all 48 months of follow-up, and 28% were abstinent for the six-month period prior to follow-up. Fifty-four percent of the clients were not in any form of remission at the four-year follow-up.

The next uproar around moderate drinking followed the publication of an article by Pendery et al. (1982). They reported that the patients in the Sobell and Sobell (1973a, 1973b, 1976) study who received training in moderate drinking did not fare as well as reported in those reports (and also in the Caddy et al. {1978} third-year evaluation). Pendery et al. (1982) reported that "most subjects trained to do controlled drinking failed from the outset to drink safely" (p. 169).

A great amount of discussion on the specifics of the Sobell and Sobell and Pendery et al. reports has been published over the ensuing years (for a small sampling see Cook, 1985, 1989; Maltzman, 1984, 1989; Marlatt, 1983; Peele, 1983; Sobell & Sobell, 1984a, 1984b, 1989; Walker & Roach, 1984; Wallace, 1990). Sobell and Sobell (1984b) themselves directly addressed issues raised by the Pendery et al. (1982) article. In addition to providing a detailed response, Sobell and Sobell (1984b) went on to conceptualize the controversy on moderate drinking as reflecting a scientific revolution that "derived less from controlled-drinking research than from the lack of support for conventional wisdom" (p. 413) regarding the nature and treatment of alcohol problems.

It is beyond the scope of the present article to critique in detail the debate surrounding the Sobell and Sobell research. The interested reader is best advised to consult the central data-based papers surrounding the study (Caddy et al., 1978; Pendery et al., 1982; Sobell & Sobell, 1973a, 1973b, 1976). However, several points warrant mention. First, a limiting feature of the Pendery et al. (1982) article is the absence of data on the comparison group of subjects who did not receive training in drinking moderation. Thus, it is not possible to report on how these two treatment approaches–relatively speaking–impacted on the posttreatment functioning of these alcoholic clients. Debate ensues on this issue (see Baker, 1989; Maltzman, 1989; and Sobell & Sobell, 1989). Second, several independent inquiries (e.g., Dickens, Doob, Warwick, & Winegard, 1982; Trachtenberg, 1984) have been conducted and each has vindicated the conduct of the Sobell and Sobell study (see Sobell and Sobell, 1989). Finally, and this perhaps is the most important point, there has been the strong temptation among many to view the Sobell and Sobell and Pendery et al. reports independent of a much larger existing body of research on moderate drinking approaches (for reviews of this broader base of research, see Miller & Hester, 1980, and Rosenberg, 1993).

Before leaving this overview of historical highlights, several other comments are in order. First, additional research on the topic of moderate drinking outcomes among alcohol dependent individuals continues to appear (e.g., Helzer, Robins, Taylor, Carey, Miller, Combs-Orme, & Farmer, 1985; Elal-Lawrence, Slade, & Dewey, 1986; Nordstrom & Berglund, 1987), with some studies involving long-term patient follow-ups. Further, there is no indication that interest in this area of research will dissipate. Second, reference must be made to a large body of research that addresses moderate drinking training among persons with low to moderate levels of alcohol dependence (reviewed by Hester & Miller, 1989, and Miller & Hester, 1980). The treatment outcomes found with this population of drinkers have been particularly impressive and reflect the importance of looking for ways of identifying which persons with drinking problems will respond best to particular treatment interventions.

## CURRENT STATUS REGARDING DRINKING MODERATION TREATMENTS

This analysis of the current status of moderate drinking treatments will revolve around two topics. The first concerns the viability of moderate drinking treatment approaches as a contemporary therapeutic strategy for persons with alcohol use disorders. The second topic is whether research on moderate drinking has helped or hindered progress in the treatment of alcohol problems.

The response to the first issue–on the viability of moderate drinking training–is that moderate drinking treatments indeed are a viable treatment modality. On one level it can be viewed as viable because moderate drinking outcomes are documented phenomena across a range of persons with alcohol use disorders, including severely dependent alcoholics. Riley, Sobell, Leo, Sobell, and Klajner (1987) found in a review of 68 treatment outcome studies published between 1978-1983 that 50% of the studies reported nonproblem drinking outcomes. However, having noted that moderate drinking outcomes do occur, it is equally if not more important to determine the predictability of such outcomes. The answer to this question introduces some qualifiers. Specifically, moderate drinking treatments geared toward populations of low to moderate severity alcohol abusers predictably yield high rates of remission of heavy drinking and drinking problems (Hester & Miller, 1989; Miller & Hester, 1980). In fact, moderate drinking interventions with low to moderate severity alcohol abusers may be the treatment of choice.

Stable moderate outcomes among severely dependent alcoholics have been less common. When they have been observed they generally have occurred following participation in treatments focused on abstinence, which of course provide no training in or encouragement of moderate drinking. The most prominent study on specifically training alcoholics to moderate their drinking (Sobell & Sobell, 1973a, 1973b, 1976) found superior outcomes among the patients receiving moderate drinking training, compared to those who received an abstinence-based treatment. While further data on the moderate drinking subjects in the Sobell and Sobell study have been provided (Pendery et al., 1982), those data shed no light on comparative effectiveness of treatment interventions for alcohol abusers because no data were provided by Pendery et al. (1982) for the control group. Indeed, there has been remarkably little research comparing moderate drinking and abstinence treatments for persons with alcohol use disorders. Sobell and Sobell (1973a, 1973b, 1976), studying an alcoholic population, and Sanchez-Craig and Lei (1986), studying a population of alcohol abusers, are notable exceptions to this state of affairs.

It is perhaps most accurate to assert that at this point in time there exists no ideal treatment of choice that reliably yields positive outcomes among alcoholic clients. A recent review of the literature published between 1978 and 1983 concluded that "treatments for alcohol problems with demonstrated enduring effectiveness do not exist, regardless of treatment orientations or treatment goals" (Riley et al., 1987, p. 107). This sobering finding, unfortunately, is not inconsistent with other reviews of alcoholism treatment over the years (e.g., Emrick, 1974, 1975; Miller & Hester, 1980). Research has suggested, however, that specific treatments geared toward specific subgroups of persons with alcohol use disorders may exhibit uniquely positive outcomes, and it is in this context that all treatments–including moderate drinking approaches–remain potentially viable in the clinician's armamentarium (as an example, see the treatment matching research by Kadden, Cooney, Getter, & Litt, 1989).

A second current status issue concerns the question of whether research on moderate drinking treatments and outcomes has helped or hindered progress in the treatment of alcohol problems. Overall it appears that the research on moderate drinking has produced several positive outcomes.

One important positive outcome is the increased attention that has been focused on the assessment and evaluation of treatment outcomes, including the reliability and validity of self-reports. This in turn has engendered a greater specification of the nature of posttreatment use of alcohol among persons treated for alcohol problems. Much of this increased focus, admittedly, has been a result of skepticism of reports of moderate drinking outcomes. Hopefully, this increased focus on moderate drinking outcomes will generalize to the assessment of all client outcomes, regardless of whether the outcome is described as remission through abstinence or moderate drinking or as nonremission (i.e., some or no improvement).

Having identified this increased evaluation of posttreatment alcohol use as a positive outcome of research on moderate drinking, a coinciding downside also needs to be mentioned. Specifically, along with the increased focus on alcohol intake and related symptomology has been a corresponding decrease in attention on other important areas of life functioning, including family/marital relationships, work performance, self-esteem, and mood/affect, among others. It is not that these domains are not being assessed, but rather that these data are not being viewed with the same attention given to drinking behavior. These domains of life functioning are of critical importance in providing an indication of overall life health posttreatment, as described in more detail by Pattison (1966) and Maisto and McCollam (1980). The tunnel-vision developing on alcohol intake–to the exclusion of other important life health dimensions–is discussed elsewhere by Heather (1989).

Returning to benefits of moderate drinking research, a second positive outcome has been an increasing recognition of and appreciation for the varied paths to remission that can be followed by persons experiencing alcohol use disorders (as described by, among others, Vaillant, 1983). These paths to recovery could include remission that involves participation in self-help groups but in the absence of formal treatment (e.g., attending meetings of Alcoholics Anonymous only) or could involve the influence of no formal external interventions whatsoever (e.g., spontaneous remission or natural recovery). These latter paths to recovery have been investigated by Tuchfeld (1981) and more recently in research being conducted by Sobell, Sobell, and Toneatto (1991). Data that describe differing courses of recovery after experiencing an alcohol problem (whether they involve treatment or result in abstinence versus moderate drinking) may be useful in developing more effective and better individualized treatments for the range of individuals experiencing problems with alcohol.

Finally, a third benefit of research on moderate drinking has been increasing awareness of the role of client goals regarding remission of their drinking problem. Research focusing on this important area (including Booth, Dale, & Ansari, 1984; Elal-Lawrence et al., 1986; and Orford & Keddie, 1986) has provided indications that there are advantages to allowing clients to identify and pursue their treatment goals. Similarly, Sanchez-Craig and Lei (1986) have described some disadvantages to arbitrarily assigning clients to a particular treatment objective (they randomly assigned problem drinkers to either a moderate drinking treatment goal or to an abstinence treatment goal). The issue of client preferences and motivations has been thoughtfully pursued in more detail by Miller (1985, 1987).

There are ways in which discourse on moderate drinking research has not been productive for the field. In some cases this has been reflected in the tendency to take a particular research report or particular clinical impression and generalize it far beyond its limitations. As an example, the Sobell and Sobell (1973, 1976) and Pendery et al. (1982) reports are but a few among a much larger group of studies on moderate drinking treatments, yet they have received a much greater (perhaps disproportionate) amount of attention. A consequence of such extrapolation is that one's awareness and perception can become focused in ways that preclude consideration of the broader array of knowledge available and questions unanswered regarding the nature of drinking problems and their resolution. Not surprisingly, the heated manner in which some of these issues have been debated has not provided a productive forum for moving forward on commonly-held objectives regarding the resolution of alcohol problems.

Before closing this section on the current status of moderate drinking research, some attention should be placed on the gap between clinical practice and clinical research. That such a gap exists is not a new insight in the alcohol field, nor is it unique to the current controversy on drinking goals and drinking outcomes. And the gaps that exist are not one-way. In some cases, the gaps are from research to practice, such as the lack of utilization of treatment techniques that are supported by research findings (see Miller & Hester, 1986). In other cases, gaps are from practice to research, such as researchers not attending to practitioners' knowledge and inputs regarding clinical phenomena or research questions of particular relevance to them. Researchers could profit by consulting more with clinicians in identifying critical research topics. It will benefit all in the field if we are able to bridge the gap between research and practice and start to move, in the words of Johns (1988), from deadlock to wedlock–or at least something analogous that permits productive communication. Strategies for enhancing interaction between research and practice have been discussed in more detail elsewhere by Ogborne (1988) and Phillips (1989).

## *SOME DIRECTIONS FOR FUTURE RESEARCH*

There are many directions for future research on moderate drinking, and only a handful will be presented here. Several of these lines of future research have been introduced in comments made earlier in this article.

One area needing attention is operationalizing terms such as problem drinking, alcohol abuse, alcoholism, and alcohol dependence. Particular further attention might be placed on distinguishing between abuse and dependence on alcohol, given the pivotal role this distinction has held in discussions on treatment goals. Some progress was made in this area with the publication of the third edition of the *Diagnostic and Statistical Manual of the Mental Disorders* (DSM-III) (APA, 1980). Despite problems in the conceptualization of abuse and dependence (see Rounsaville, 1987), the distinction did provide useful options (and opportunities) in diagnosis and treatment. The revised third edition (DSM-III-R) (APA, 1987) relegated the alcohol abuse diagnosis to a residual status and effectively eliminated the abuse-dependence distinction many had found useful. Early indications are that DSM-IV will reinstate this distinction between abuse and dependence (see Nathan, 1991, for the current status of substance use disorders in DSM-IV). Further research on this classification system, as well as research using other systems, will serve the important purpose of better defining the nature of alcohol problems and improving communication.

Research also is needed on defining outcome. The definitions used to define abstinence, moderate drinking, and other categories of outcome have varied considerably from study to study. This makes comparisons between research reports difficult if not impossible. Advancements in understanding treatment outcomes will benefit from a more uniform use of outcome categories. Relatedly, additional attention needs to be placed on assessing other domains of life functioning that can be enhanced by treatment interventions, such as physical and psychological health, work status, family functioning, and the like.

More research is needed to specify the role of alcohol dependence severity and the likelihood of achieving remission of alcohol problems through drinking moderation. It has been hypothesized that the likelihood of achieving a posttreatment pattern of moderate drinking is inversely related to severity of alcohol dependence. However, research on this topic has been mixed, and several studies have not indicated this hypothesized relationship (e.g., Elal-Lawrence et al., 1986; Orford & Keddie, 1986; Rychtarik, Foy, Scott, Lokey, & Prue, 1985).

Finally, research should address further the areas of client choice/preference and the varied paths to recovery alcohol abusers may follow. Some work in these areas, cited earlier, has already been conducted. The accumulation of additional knowledge in these domains will be of much potential benefit in understanding the processes involved in recovering from alcohol problems and could make helpful contributions to efforts to match clients to treatments.

## CONCLUSIONS

Research on moderate drinking among persons with alcohol use disorders has been controversial but nevertheless has extended knowledge about alcohol problems and their treatment. In this assessment of the current status of moderate drinking research, it is concluded, first, that moderate drinking treatments indeed are a viable treatment approach for some alcohol abusers, and, second, that research in this area has advanced and will continue to advance progress in the treatment of alcohol problems. Steps need to be initiated by both researchers and practitioners to bridge the gap between them. In the absence of such efforts, progress in the treatment of alcohol use disorders will be slow and tedious.

## REFERENCES

American Psychiatric Association (APA). (1980). *Diagnostic and statistical manual of mental disorders* (Third Ed.). Washington, DC: APA.

American Psychiatric Association (APA). (1987). *Diagnostic and statistical manual of mental disorders* (Revised Third Ed.). Washington, DC: APA.

Armor, D.J., Polich, J.M., & Stambul, H.B. (1976). *Alcoholism and treatment.* Santa Monica: Rand Corporation.

Armor, D. J., Stambul, H. B., & Polich, J. M. (1977). The "Rand Report": Some comments and a response. *Journal of Studies on Alcohol, 38,* 179-193.

Baker, T. (1989). An open letter to Journal readers. *Journal of Studies on Alcohol, 50,* 481-483.

Block, M. A. (1962). Comment on the article by D. L. Davies. *Quarterly Journal of Studies on Alcohol, 24,* 114-117.

Blume, S. (1977). The "Rand Report": Some comments and a response. *Journal of Studies on Alcohol, 38,* 163-168.

Booth, P.G., Dale, B., & Ansari, J. (1984). Problem drinkers' goal choice and treatment outcome: A preliminary study. *Addictive Behaviors, 9,* 357-364.

Caddy, G. R., Addington, H. J., & Perkins, D. (1978). Individualized behavior therapy for alcoholics: A third year independent double-blind follow-up. *Behaviour Research and Therapy, 16,* 345-362.

Cohen, M., Liebson, I. A., & Faillace, L. A. (1972). A technique for establishing controlled drinking in chronic alcoholics. *Diseases of the Nervous System, 33,* 46-49.

Cohen, M., Liebson, I.A., Faillace, L. A., & Speers, W. (1971). Alcoholism: Controlled drinking and incentives for abstinence. *Psychological Reports, 28,* 575-580.

Cook, D. R. (1985). Craftsman versus professional: Analysis of the controlled drinking controversy. *Journal of Studies on Alcohol, 46,* 433-442.

Cook, D. R. (1989). A reply to Maltzman. *Journal of Studies on Alcohol, 50,* 484-486.

Davies, D.L. (1962). Normal drinking in recovered alcohol addicts. *Quarterly Journal of Studies on Alcohol, 23,* 94-104.

Dickens, B.M., Doob, A.N., Warwick, O.H., & Winegard, W. C. (1982). *Report of the committee of enquiry into allegations concerning Drs. Linda and Mark Sobell.* Toronto: Addiction Research Foundation.

Edwards, G. (1985a). Paradigm shift or change in ownership? The conceptual significance of D.L. Davies's classic paper. *Drug and Alcohol Dependence, 15,* 19-35.

Edwards, G. (1985b). A later follow-up of a classic case series: D.L. Davies's 1962 report and its significance for the present. *Journal of Studies on Alcohol, 46,* 181-190.

Elal-Lawrence, G., Slade, P. D., & Dewey, M. E. (1986). Predictors of outcome type in treated problem drinkers. *Journal of Studies on Alcohol, 47,* 41-47.

Emrick, C. D. (1974). A review of psychologically oriented treatment of alcoholism. I. The use and interrelationships of outcome criteria and drinking behavior following treatment. *Quarterly Journal of Studies on Alcohol, 35,* 523-549.

Emrick, C. D. (1975). A review of psychologically oriented treatment of alcoholism. II. The relative effectiveness of different treatment approaches and the effectiveness of treatment versus no treatment. *Quarterly Journal of Studies on Alcohol, 36,* 88-108.

Emrick, C. D., & Stilson, D. W. (1977). The "Rand Report": Some comments and a response. *Journal of Studies on Alcohol, 38,* 152-163.

Engle, K. B., & Williams, T. K. (1972). Effect of an ounce of vodka on alcoholics' desire for alcohol. *Quarterly Journal of Studies on Alcohol, 33,* 1099-1105.

Heather, N. (1989). Controlled drinking treatment: Where do we stand today? In T. Loberg, W. R. Miller, P. E. Nathan, & G. A. Marlatt (Eds.), *Addictive behaviors: Prevention and early intervention* (pp. 31-50). Amsterdam: Swets & Zeitlinger.

Heather, N., & Robertson, I.H. (1981). *Controlled drinking.* London: Methuen.

Helzer, J.E., Robins, L.N., Taylor, J.R., Carey, K., Miller, R. H., Combs-Orme, T., & Farmer, A. (1985). The extent of long-term moderate drinking among alcoholics discharged from medical and psychiatric treatment facilities. *New England Journal of Medicine, 312,* 1678-1682.

Hester, R. K., & Miller, W. R. (1989). Self-control training. In R. K. Hester & W. R. Miller (Eds.), *Handbook of alcoholism treatment approaches* (pp. 141-149). New York: Pergamon.

Johns, A. (1988). The alliance between research and clinical practice in drug dependence—wedlock or deadlock? *British Journal of Addiction, 83,* 725-727.

Kadden, R. M., Cooney, N. L., Getter, H., & Litt, M. D. (1989). Matching alcoholics to coping skills or interactional therapies: Posttreatment results. *Journal of Consulting and Clinical Psychology, 57,* 698-704.

Lemere, F. (1963). Comment on the article by D. L. Davies. *Quarterly Journal of Studies on Alcohol, 24,* 727-728.

Lolli, G. (1963). Comment on the article by D. L. Davies. *Quarterly Journal of Studies on Alcohol, 24,* 326-330.

Lovibond, S.H., & Caddy, G.R. (1970). Discriminated aversive control in the moderation of alcoholics' drinking behavior. *Behavior Therapy, 1,* 437-444.

Maisto, S. A., & McCollam, J. B. (1980). The use of multiple measures of life health to assess alcohol treatment outcome: A review and critique. L. C. Sobell, M. B. Sobell, & E. Ward (Eds.), *Evaluating alcohol and drug abuse treatment effectiveness: Recent advances.* New York: Pergamon, 1980.

Maltzman, I. (1984). More on: "Controlled drinking versus abstinence: Where do we go from here?" *Bulletin of the Society of Psychologists in Addictive Behaviors, 3,* 71-73.

Maltzman, I. (1989). A reply to Cook, "Craftsman versus professional: Analysis of the controlled drinking controversy." *Journal of Studies on Alcohol, 50,* 466-472.

Marlatt, G.A. (1983). The controlled-drinking controversy: A commentary. *American Psychologist, 38,* 1097-1110.

Mello, N. K., & Mendelson, J. H. (1972). Drinking patterns during work-contingent and non-contingent alcohol acquisition. *Psychosomatic Medicine, 34,* 139-164.

Miller, W.R. (1983). Controlled drinking: A history and a critical review. *Journal of Studies on Alcohol, 44,* 68-83.

Miller, W. R. (1985). Motivation for treatment: A review with special emphasis on alcoholism. *Psychological Bulletin, 98,* 84-107.

Miller, W. R. (1987). Motivation and treatment goals. *Drugs & Society, 1,* 133-151.

Miller, W.R., & Hester, R.K. (1980). Treating the problem drinker: Modern approaches. In W.R. Miller (Ed.), *The addictive behaviors: Treatment of alcoholism, drug abuse, smoking, and obesity* (pp. 11-141). Elmsford, NY: Pergamon.

Miller, W. R., & Hester, R. K. (1986). The effectiveness of alcoholism treatment: What research reveals. In W. R. Miller & N. Heather (Eds.), *Treating addictive behaviors: Processes of change* (pp. 121-174). New York: Plenum Press.

Myerson, D. J. (1963). Comment on the article by D. L. Davies. *Quarterly Journal of Studies on Alcohol, 24,* 325.

Nathan, P. E. (1991). Substance use disorders in the DSM-IV. *Journal of Abnormal Psychology, 100,* 356-361.

National Institute on Alcohol Abuse and Alcoholism (NIAAA). (1990). *Seventh Special Report to the U.S. Congress on Alcohol and Health.* Rockville, MD: DHHS.

Nordstrom, G., & Berglund, M. (1987). A prospective study of successful long-term adjustment in alcohol dependence: Social drinking versus abstinence. *Journal of Studies on Alcohol, 48,* 95-103.

Ogborne, A. C. (1988). Bridging the gap between the two cultures of alcoholism research and treatment. *British Journal of Addiction, 83,* 729-733.

Orford, J., & Keddie, A. (1986). Abstinence or controlled drinking in clinical practice: Indications at initial assessment. *Addictive Behaviors, 11,* 71-86.

Pattison, E. M. (1966). A critique of alcoholism treatment concepts with special reference to abstinence. *Quarterly Journal of Studies on Alcohol, 27,* 49-71.

Pattison, E.M. (1976). Nonabstinent drinking goals in the treatment of alcoholics. In R.J. Gibbins, Y. Israel, H. Kalant, R. E. Popham, W. Schmidt, & R. G. Smart (Eds.), *Research advances in alcohol and drug problems* (vol. 3) (pp. 401-455). New York: John Wiley & Sons.

Pattison, E.M., Headley, E.D., Gleser, G.C., & Gottschalk, L.A. (1968). Abstinence and normal drinking: An assessment of changes in drinking patterns in alcoholics after treatment. *Quarterly Journal of Studies on Alcohol, 29,* 610-633.

Peele, S. (April, 1983). Through a glass darkly. *Psychology Today,* 38-42.

Pendery, M.L., Maltzman, I.M., & West, L.J. (1982). Controlled drinking by alcoholics? New findings and a reevaluation of a major affirmative study. *Science, 217,* 169-175.

Phillips, B. N. (1989). Role of the practitioner in applying science to practice. *Professional Psychology: Research and Practice, 20,* 3-8.

Polich, J.M., Armor, D.J., & Braiker, H.B. (1981). *The course of alcoholism: Four years after treatment.* New York: Wiley.

Reinert, R.E., & Bowen, W.T. (1968). Social drinking following treatment for alcoholism. *Bulletin of the Menninger Clinic, 32,* 280-290.

Riley, D. M., Sobell, L. C., Leo, G. I., Sobell, M. B., & Klajner, F. (1987). Behavioral treatment of alcohol problems: A review and a comparison of behavioral and nonbehavioral studies. In W. M. Cox (Ed.), *Treatment and prevention of alcohol problems: A resource manual* (pp. 73-115). New York: Academic Press.

Roizen, R. (1987). The great controlled-drinking controversy. In M. Galanter (Ed.), *Recent developments in alcoholism* (pp. 245-279). New York: Plenum.

Rosenberg, H. (1993). Prediction of controlled drinking by alcoholics and problem drinkers. *Psychological Bulletin, 113,* 129-139.

Rounsaville, B. J. (1987). An evaluation of the DSM-III substance use disorders. In G. Tischler (Ed.), *Treatment and classification in psychiatry* (pp. 175-194). New York: Cambridge University Press.

Rychtarik, R. G., Foy, D. W., Scott, T., Lokey, L., & Prue, D. M. (1987). Five-six year follow-up of broadspectrum treatment for alcoholism: Effects of training controlled drinking skills. *Journal of Consulting and Clinical Psychology, 55,* 106-108.

Sanchez-Craig, M., & Lei, H. (1986). Disadvantages to imposing the goal of abstinence on problem drinkers: An empirical study. *British Journal of Addiction, 81,* 1-8.

Selzer, M. L. (1963). Comment on the article by D. L. Davies. *Quarterly Journal of Studies on Alcohol, 24,* 113-114.

Selzer, M.L., & Holloway, W.H. (1957). A follow-up of alcoholics committed to a state hospital. *Quarterly Journal of Studies on Alcohol, 18,* 98-120.

Smith, H., & Jackson, G. (1982). The Rand Report reviewed: A critical analysis. *Advances in Alcohol and Substance Abuse, 2,* 7-16.

Sobell, L. C., Sobell, M. B., & Toneatto, T. (1991). Recovery from alcohol problems without treatment. In N. Heather, W. R. Miller, & J. Greeley (Eds.), *Self-control and the addictive behaviours* (pp. 198-242). New York: Pergamon.

Sobell, M. B., & Sobell, L. C. (1973a). Individualized behavior therapy for alcoholics. *Behavior Therapy, 4*, 49-72.

Sobell, M.B., & Sobell, L.C. (1973b). Alcoholics treated by individualized behavior therapy: One-year treatment outcome. *Behaviour Research and Therapy, 11*, 599-618.

Sobell, M.B., & Sobell, L.C. (1976). Second year treatment outcome of alcoholics treated by individualized behavior therapy: Results. *Behaviour Research and Therapy, 14*, 195-215.

Sobell, M. B., & Sobell, L.C. (1984a). Under the microscope yet again: A commentary on Walker and Roach's critique of the Dickens Committee's enquiry into our research. *British Journal of Addiction, 79*, 157-168.

Sobell, M.B., & Sobell, L.C. (1984b). The aftermath of heresy: A response to Pendery et al. (1982) critique of "Individualized Behavior Therapy for Alcoholics." *Behaviour Research and Therapy, 22*, 413-440.

Sobell, M. B., & Sobell, L. C. (1989). Moratorium on Maltzman: An appeal to reason. *Journal of Studies on Alcohol, 50*, 473-480.

Tiebout, H. M. (1962). Comment on the article by D. L. Davies. *Quarterly Journal of Studies on Alcohol, 24*, 109-111.

Trachtenberg, R. L. (1984). Report of the Steering Group to the Administrator, Alcohol, Drug Abuse, and Mental Health Administration regarding its attempts to investigate allegations of scientific misconduct concerning Drs. Mark and Linda Sobell. Rockville, MD: Alcohol, Drug Abuse, and Mental Health Administration.

Tuchfeld, B. S. (1981). Spontaneous remission in alcoholics: Empirical observations and theoretical implications. *Journal of Studies on Alcohol, 42*, 626-641.

Vaillant, G. E. (1983). *The natural history of alcoholism: Causes, patterns, and paths to recovery*. Cambridge: Harvard University Press.

Walker, K. D., & Roach, C. A. (1984). A critique of the report of the Dickens' enquiry into the controlled drinking research of the Sobells. *British Journal of Addiction, 79*, 147-156.

Wallace, J. (1990). Abstinence and non-abstinence goals in treatment: A case study in the sociology of knowledge. In R. C. Engs (Ed.), *Controversies in the addiction's field* (vol. 1) (pp. 192-202). Dubuque, Iowa: Kendall/Hunt.

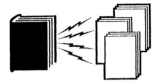

# Haworth
# DOCUMENT DELIVERY
## SERVICE
### and Local Photocopying Royalty Payment Form

This new service provides (a) a single-article order form for any article from a Haworth journal and (b) a convenient royalty payment form for local photocopying (not applicable to photocopies intended for resale).

- *Time Saving:* No running around from library to library to find a specific article.
- *Cost Effective:* All costs are kept down to a minimum.
- *Fast Delivery:* Choose from several options, including same-day FAX.
- *No Copyright Hassles:* You will be supplied by the original publisher.
- *Easy Payment:* Choose from several easy payment methods.

*Open Accounts Welcome for . . .*
- Library Interlibrary Loan Departments
- Library Network/Consortia Wishing to Provide Single-Article Services
- Indexing/Abstracting Services with Single Article Provision Services
- Document Provision Brokers and Freelance Information Service Providers

### MAIL or *FAX* THIS ENTIRE ORDER FORM TO:

Attn: **Marianne Arnold**
Haworth Document Delivery Service
The Haworth Press, Inc.
10 Alice Street
Binghamton, NY 13904-1580

or FAX: (607) 722-1424
or CALL: 1-800-3-HAWORTH
(1-800-342-9678; 9am-5pm EST)

---

PLEASE SEND ME PHOTOCOPIES OF THE FOLLOWING SINGLE ARTICLES:

1) Journal Title: _____
   Vol/Issue/Year:_____Starting & Ending Pages:_____
   Article Title:_____
   _____

2) Journal Title: _____
   Vol/Issue/Year:_____Starting & Ending Pages:_____
   Article Title:_____
   _____

3) Journal Title: _____
   Vol/Issue/Year:_____Starting & Ending Pages:_____
   Article Title:_____
   _____

4) Journal Title: _____
   Vol/Issue/Year:_____Starting & Ending Pages:_____
   Article Title:_____
   _____

**(See other side for Costs and Payment Information)**

*COSTS:* Please figure your cost to order quality copies of an article.

1. Set-up charge per article: $8.00
   ($8.00 × number of separate articles)     _____

2. Photocopying charge for each article:
   - 1-10 pages: $1.00     _____
   - 11-19 pages: $3.00     _____
   - 20-29 pages: $5.00     _____
   - 30+ pages: $2.00/10 pages     _____

3. Flexicover (optional): $2.00/article     _____

4. Postage & Handling:   US: $1.00 for the first article/
   $.50 each additional article     _____
   Federal Express: $25.00     _____
   Outside US: $2.00 for first article/
   $.50 each additional article_____

5. Same-day FAX service: $.35 per page     _____

6. Local Photocopying Royalty Payment: should you wish to copy the article yourself. Not intended for photocopies made for resale. $1.50 per article per copy (i.e. 10 articles x $1.50 each = $15.00)     _____

**GRAND TOTAL:**     _____

*METHOD OF PAYMENT:* (please check one)

❑ Check enclosed     ❑ Please ship and bill. PO # _____
(sorry we can ship and bill to bookstores only! All others must pre-pay)

❑ Charge to my credit card:   ❑ Visa;   ❑ MasterCard;   ❑ American Express;

Account Number:_____     Expiration date:_____

Signature: *X*_____     Name:  _____

Institution: _____     Address: _____

City: _____     State:_____   Zip:_____

Phone Number: _____     FAX Number: _____

## MAIL or *FAX* THIS ENTIRE ORDER FORM TO:

Attn: **Marianne Arnold**
Haworth Document Delivery Service
The Haworth Press, Inc.
10 Alice Street
Binghamton, NY 13904-1580

or **FAX:** (607) 722-1424
or **CALL:** 1-800-3-HAWORTH
(1-800-342-9678; 9am-5pm EST)